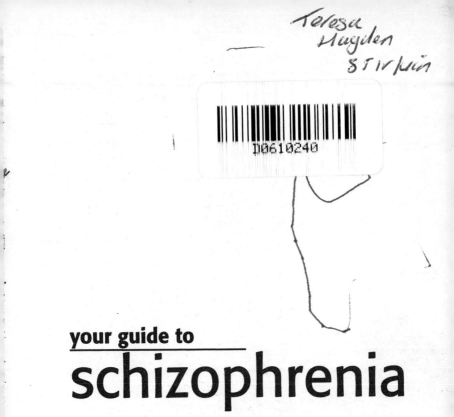

your guide to

schizophrenia

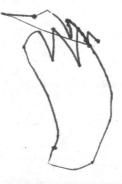

The ROYAL
SOCIETY *of*
MEDICINE

your guide to
schizophrenia

Dr Adrianne M. Reveley
MB BCH, MRC Psych

Hodder Arnold

A MEMBER OF THE HODDER HEADLINE GROUP

Orders: Please contact Bookpoint Ltd, 130 Milton Park, Abingdon, Oxon OX14 4SB. Telephone: (44) 01235 827720, Fax: (44) 01235 400454. Lines are open from 9.00 to 17.00, Monday to Saturday, with a 24-hour message answering service. You can also order through our website www.hoddereducation.com

British Library Cataloguing in Publication Data
A catalogue record for this title is available from the British Library.

ISBN-10: 0 340 92747 X
ISBN-13: 9 780340 927472
First published   2006
Impression number   10 9 8 7 6 5 4 3 2
Year   2008   2007
Copyright © 2006 Adrianne Reveley

Typeset by Servis Filmsetting Limited, Longsight, Manchester. Printed in Great Britain for Hodder Arnold, a division of Hodder Headline, an Hachette Livre UK Company, 338 Euston Road, London NW1 3BH, by Cox & Wyman Ltd, Reading, Berkshire.

Every effort has been made to trace copyright for material used in this book. The authors and publishers would be happy to make arrangements with any holder of copyright whom it has not been possible to trace successfully by the time of going to press.

The publisher has used its best endeavours to ensure that the URLs for external websites referred to in this book are correct and active at the time of going to press. However, the publisher and the author have no responsibility for the websites and can make no guarantee that a site will remain live or that the content will remain relevant, decent or appropriate.

Hachette's policy is to use papers that are natural, renewable and recyclable products and made from wood grown in sustainable forests. The logging and manufacturing processes are expected to conform to the environmental regulations of the country of origin

Contents

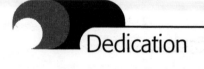

Dedication

To all my patients and their carers from whom I
have learnt so much. Their courageous struggle
with the illness has been a constant inspiration.

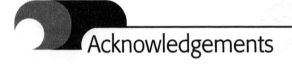

Acknowledgements

I would like to express my thanks to members of the Rethink National Advice Team; Mary Teasdale, Gabrielle Ayerst, Ann Baldwin and Gerry Horner for their help with this book.

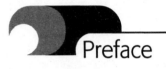

Preface

This new book, published in partnership with the Royal Society of Medicine, provides detailed, useful and up-to-date information on schizophrenia. It contains expert yet user-friendly advice, with such useful features as:

Key Terms: demystifying the jargon
Questions and Answers: answering the burning questions
Myths and Facts: debunking the misconceptions
My Experience: how it feels to live with, or care for someone, with this condition.

Bearing the hallmark of excellence and accessibility that characterizes the work of the Royal Society of Medicine, this important guide will enable you and your family to gain some control over the way your schizophrenia is managed by being better informed.

Peter Richardson
Director of Publications
Royal Society of Medicine

Introduction

New and better insights into the cause and treatment of schizophrenia have occurred over the past ten years. The changes in the brain accompanying schizophrenia are better understood; we have seen the development of better services for the mentally ill, improved psychotherapy techniques, new and better medication, and other exciting developments which have all contributed to a much more positive view of schizophrenia, and a realistic chance for lasting recovery.

However, the more positive attitude in the scientific/psychiatric world has not been mirrored by knowledge of, and attitudes to, schizophrenia by the general public. While the man or woman in the street has a fairly accurate concept of conditions such as HIV/AIDS, or Alzheimer's disease, for example, he/she draws a blank when it comes to schizophrenia. Part of the problem is that facts about mental illness are not well taught in schools, and even medical students or budding GPs do not have to study mental illness in depth. For this reason, most people get their ideas about schizophrenia from media stories, but unfortunately the media focus is on extreme incidents, such as a random, motiveless attack on a stranger by a schizophrenic patient. These extreme examples skew our thinking and generate misinformation and intense anxiety. Poor understanding is associated with a number of adverse reactions such as fear, rejection and even denial that the illness exists at all.

Schizophrenia usually affects young people at the start of their lives, and it can last a lifetime – these are further reasons for anxiety and fear. Our ignorance about schizophrenia allows powerful myths and old ideas to persist, and these are often damaging to families and frightening to people with the illness, and lead to stigma. People shy away from the diagnosis; they may deny their problems, blame their families or blame the doctor. But hiding the illness away feeds into the vicious circle of ignorance, fear and greater stigma.

This book aims to improve current knowledge about the causes and symptoms of schizophrenia and to outline the best way to achieve recovery, as well as debunking myths and showing how erroneous ideas arose in the past. Up-to-date, accurate information about schizophrenia can be important and immensely reassuring, although knowledge about the biological basis of schizophrenia may actually increase stigma unless it is also emphasized that there are helpful treatments and positive outcomes. Full or substantial recovery is a realistic aspiration for almost everyone affected by schizophrenia. Now we really know and can explain what happens in the brain when someone hallucinates. We know and can explain the principal ways in which medicines work. We have better ideas about how people with the illness, and their families and carers, can best be helped, and we know that some people can recover and live normal lives. We have better opportunities for tackling the illness early on and preventing some of the long-term consequences. Hopefully the information in this book will go some way to counter the myths and provide useful indicators on the pathway to recovery.

CHAPTER

1

What is schizophrenia?

Schizophrenia is the formal psychiatric name for a recognized mental disorder with defined characteristics. It is not a loose or ill-defined term, despite the way it is so often used by the media, or in general conversation.

Schizophrenia is an illness which happens to affect the brain. It usually comes on in early adulthood, at around the time that the brain has finished maturing, and often becomes a **chronic**, long-term problem, affecting all aspects of a person's life. The fact that schizophrenia can last a lifetime, together with mistaken ideas about people with schizophrenia being violent, and general ignorance about the causes and symptoms, leads to considerable anxiety and fear when the diagnosis is mentioned.

Schizophrenia is one of a group of illnesses called 'psychoses', so called because, at some stage of the illness, **psychosis** may occur. The

chronic (of illness)
Of long duration and recurrent; may be mild in degree. Often mistakenly thought to mean 'serious'.

schizophrenia
A psychiatrically defined mental disorder characterized by positive (psychotic) and negative (motivational) symptoms, generally treated with antipsychotic medication.

my experience

Harvey was a happy child, good at his school work with lots of friends. We had no worries about him, unlike Milly (Harvey's sister) who was always difficult. Harvey did well enough in his A levels – maybe he could have tried harder, but he went on to university. He chose somewhere miles away, which his mother and I took to be a sign of wanting to fly the nest.

The first sign we had that there were any problems at all were towards the end of Harvey's first year, when we had a call from one of his flatmates, saying that he was behaving strangely, and refusing to leave his room. Harvey wouldn't come to the phone. We left for Scotland immediately, but when we got there, Harvey had run away without any money and wearing just a T-shirt. We searched the neighbourhood. Harvey turned up two days later, so frightened he was almost incoherent. He was talking about 'elite forces' watching him and following him, because he could control the weather and had other special talents, and there was something about preventing world disasters. His mother and I were horrified, and got him admitted straightaway to a local mental hospital. He was diagnosed with probable schizophrenia and put on medication.

Within three weeks of starting the medication Harvey was well enough to leave hospital and come home. He was really back to himself by then, although he was pretty shaken by it all. We were told he should stay on the medication for at least a year, which he did. That was four years ago now. Harvey has managed to get a degree since then, at a university closer to home, and he's currently working in our local bookshop while he decides what career path to take. He seems absolutely fine, but we have a lot of unanswered questions.

psychosis (plural 'psychoses')
A mental disorder involving the individual in extreme distortions of thought which lead to a lack of contact with reality. The individual will often have no insight into this process.

core feature of psychosis is a permanent or intermittent loss of contact with reality, which is thought to be due to a malfunction in the part of the brain that governs sensation and emotion (the temporo-parietal/limbic area). Errors in this part of the brain lead to problems in our ability to process sensory information from the outside world, and to distinguish between our own inner thoughts and feelings, and the experiences we have which come from outside ourselves. This is because when someone becomes **psychotic**, their brain loses its ability to tell between perceptions it has generated itself, from those that it has received from outside the body. When this happens, thoughts may be misinterpreted as voices, or imaginary images may be seen as visions. Similar **hallucinations** may occur involving sense of smell or touch. Sometimes individuals believe that there are strange smells around them, or that they themselves smell, or may feel touched by an unseen hand, even in the genital area, which can lead to complaints that they are being interfered with. Auditory hallucinations are the most common. **Delusions** may also develop; these are fixed, false beliefs that have no basis in reality. The person with psychosis may also develop problems with their thinking, so that their thought processes become disorganized and lack logical coherence.

Psychosis occurs in several different conditions, not only schizophrenia, but there are also other problems associated with schizophrenia which make it unique. There is often a slow development of difficulties such as social withdrawal, lack of motivation, loss of interest in friends, studies or work, deterioration in hygiene or grooming, unusual behaviour, or outbursts of anger. In effect, the person stops leading their normal life and no longer behaves in their own normal fashion. If this happens in adolescence, family members may think it is a 'phase'. It is only when some of the other symptoms of schizophrenia become apparent, that the behaviour is recognized as a mental illness.

psychotic
This is a technical psychiatric term and does not mean 'dangerous' as is commonly thought.

hallucination
A false sensory experience with no basis in reality. Senses involved can include: auditory (hearing voices), visual, taste, smell or touch.

delusion
A false belief which is firmly held.

Q What is psychosis?

A Psychosis refers to a mental state in which the person experiences a constellation of subjective experiences which have no basis in reality. When a person is psychotic, the usual sensory information received by the brain (sight, hearing, touch, smell) can be misinterpreted, leading to hallucinations (of hearing, sight, touch or smell). Auditory hallucinations are

A the most common. There may also be fixed, false beliefs (delusions) and/or disorganized thought processes with loosening of logical associations or train of thought.

Sometimes the onset of schizophrenia is associated with a sudden and dramatic psychosis, with a previously normal individual changing over a number of days or weeks and starting to behave in a strange or bizarre fashion. Sometimes schizophrenia comes on gradually over months or even a number of years.

In addition to the delusions and hallucinations associated with psychosis, people with schizophrenia may lose energy, initiative and motivation. Sometimes mental abilities, skills or intellectual 'sharpness' gradually decline. Social skills are very often lost. These changes are very frightening and bewildering both for the person concerned, and for those close to them.

Q What is happening to the brain when psychosis develops?

A The brain is said to be the most complicated thing on the planet. There are about 100,000 million brain cells with connections between them as complicated as the world's entire telecommunications system. When the connections in the limbic area of the brain are faulty, errors develop in the ability to process information about the outside world and about ourselves, and this is known as 'psychosis'.

The symptoms of schizophrenia

myth
Schizophrenia is just 'hearing voices'.

fact
One of the traditional ideas about schizophrenia, that it is simply 'hearing voices', is far from the truth. Many people hear voices without having schizophrenia or psychosis at all. It is, for instance, fairly common to hear your name called on waking up or going to sleep. For schizophrenia to be diagnosed, there must be a specific pattern of behavioural or life difficulties, as well as psychosis, which *could* be manifest by hearing voices, but this is just one possible psychotic symptom among many.

People with schizophrenia may experience a considerable range of symptoms associated with the malfunctioning of the brain. It is often said that one person with the illness may not share a single symptom with another. However, overall, the symptoms and problems of the illness fall into two basic groups: **psychotic symptoms** (known as 'positive' symptoms because they appear to be experiences or attributes that are 'added on' to the person), and **negative symptoms** (so-called because they represent features that are lost by the person). Negative symptoms include problems with motivation, energy and drive, as well as the ability to think and plan. In addition, people who are developing, or who already have schizophrenia often become depressed, and depressive or suicidal symptoms also form part of the illness.

Positive symptoms

The positive symptoms are not specific to schizophrenia; because they are, in effect, psychotic symptoms, they occur in other psychoses as well (e.g. bipolar disorder or psychotic depression). Positive symptoms are most often seen in the **acute** stages of the illness (sometimes called **florid** stages). They can reflect distortions of reality experienced through any or all the senses of the body, and may come on gradually, or quite suddenly.

Positive or psychotic symptoms are the most amenable to medication. In about 80 per cent of people these symptoms will lessen dramatically, or often disappear, with the right medication.

Hallucinations

Auditory hallucinations are the most frequent and are most often experienced as voices, and may be heard in the second person (e.g.

psychotic ('positive') symptoms
The normal senses (hearing, vision, touch, smell, taste) may appear faulty due to a failure of the brain to distinguish its own internal activity from things happening in the outside world.

negative symptoms
These symptoms represent loss of function. Personality characteristics may be lost or flattened. Initiative, energy and motivation are reduced, social skills lost, emotions dulled or altered, and the individual tends to withdraw from society.

acute
Serious and arising quickly.

florid
Strongly in evidence and not hidden. Usually applied to psychotic symptoms.

another person saying 'You smell', 'You are a fag') and occasionally voices can command the person to do something (e.g. 'Jump off that bridge', 'Walk in front of that car'). Third person hallucinations, in which the person hears two or more voices discussing among themselves, or commenting on the person's behaviour, are thought to be more particular to schizophrenia than to the other psychoses (e.g. 'He's a fag. Yes, look at him mincing along' or 'She's a slut isn't she? Let's punish her for it. Yes, let's punish her'). Auditory hallucinations often have a 'worst fear' quality.

Sometimes people feel as though their own thoughts are audible, and can be heard by other people, or are being broadcast aloud. They may feel as though other people's thoughts have been inserted into their own minds, or their thoughts have been taken away by someone else.

Hallucinations in the other senses also occur. Sometimes people with schizophrenia experience 'tactile' hallucinations (hallucinations of touch) and may feel that they are being pushed, or held down. Visual hallucinations can appear as visions of strange people, or fantastic objects, or sometimes as simple 'grid' patterns or a regular pattern of dots superimposed over the field of vision (not to be confused with 'floaters' in the eyes!). Occasionally people will report that certain colours appear much brighter than they should do, or details will 'spring out' of the background, such as the pattern of the grain in a wooden table. Hallucinations of smell are less common, but can be intensely distressing. People may feel that they themselves smell, and may go to great lengths to avoid other people.

Joe was brought to hospital after being found running down the hard shoulder of the busy M2. He said he was being followed by aliens in space ships, and they were communicating with him by 'blasting' his brain with noise, and he felt his brain was being eaten alive. Joe described a sensation of terrible physical pain, fear and impending doom; he couldn't cope and felt he had to run away. Up to a few weeks before this incident, Joe was quite well.

Delusions

Delusional ideas may develop. These are fixed or unshakeable beliefs formed on the basis of the psychotic person's own altered reality. These beliefs may not correspond at all to the world as other people see it. It is easy to understand how this happens. If internal reality is altered, and the person with psychosis cannot tell the difference between something they have heard, or something they have thought, they may believe that they are actually being controlled or pursued by something else, like another person, or by an alien, or a machine. The sound of a helicopter overhead may terrify them and mean to them that they are being followed. If the negative thoughts about ourselves, that we all have from time to time, are misinterpreted as someone else's negative comments (which can happen in psychosis), then it can seem to the person with psychosis that he or she is being picked on or persecuted. Sometimes delusional ideas are grandiose; the person may believe that they are able to control the world, or the weather, or that they are a god.

Sometimes quite arbitrary events or circumstances may be seen as significant – for example a green van passing on the road is seen as a 'sign'. Delusional ideas are not open to reassurance or rational argument.

Thought disorder

thought disorder
Present when there are marked abnormalities in the form and flow of thought.

Occasionally, in severe cases of psychosis, something known as **thought disorder** develops, where language loses its syntax, and the person appears to invent new words and phrases. The box below gives an example of 'thought disorder'.

information

'I find human witness verified substantiated as actual material human endouvair and a new revelation of sex practice, in this it would seem the incorporation of voice barrage plays an important part, here we have it 24 hours a day aaand this has carried on for the past ten years it would only cover one period, along with the body-head Activation by Radio-Active methods, it has even been developed and used by business sales, even to voice head communication method of everything possible, to even include this type of distance sex practice both seses taking part the single being freely induced to be the Incubus and Succubus, or Induced until self-concience . . .'

(Reprinted from *Clinical Psychiatry*, eds Slater and Roth Williams & Wilkins Baltimore, 3rd edition 1969)

A case history

The following vignette illustrates visual hallucinations, but also that the diagnosis of schizophrenia involves more than just having hallucinations; it also includes a range of tell-tale signs of social deterioration. This case vignette also illustrates the tendency of schizophrenia to occur at times of social stress, particularly if the person feels in some way 'different' or 'alienated'. (This will be discussed further in Chapter 3.)

my experience

Jerome, who was of part-Russian origin, was deaf from birth. He was brought up in a very supportive and successful (hearing) family and communicated well through sign language and lip-reading. He was a gifted artist and did well at a specialized school for the deaf, and went on to an art college. Jerome had some difficulties fitting in to the hearing world at college and said he felt 'different' or 'alienated', although he did manage to form a relationship with a girl.

During his second term at college, Jerome gradually started to become more withdrawn and 'distant', with outbursts of irritability. His painting gradually became more disorganized and he would concentrate on detail, rather than the overall composition. He stopped keeping regular hours, and was often up all night, and asleep all day. He split up with his girlfriend and spent long periods alone in his room. His personal care deteriorated and he started to behave oddly. He would place objects around the room in strange and 'significant' places. For example, he would leave an atlas opened to a particular page, showing Russia, on his flat-mate's bed.

Jerome was finally admitted to a specialized mental health unit for the deaf, where he was diagnosed with schizophrenia. Jerome told the doctors that he was hallucinating a small man who popped up out of drawers when he opened them, or peeped around doors, and the little man would sign obscene and insulting things to him, telling him that he was 'gay' because he had a male flat-mate, and that his flat-mate planned to have him deported to Russia. Jerome responded well to medication and he recovered completely, although he went on to have several further episodes of illness at times of stress in his life.

Negative symptoms

Many people say that the negative symptoms of schizophrenia are more difficult to cope with than the psychotic/positive symptoms. These symptoms are certainly the hardest to treat, although some medication, particularly the new atypical antipsychotics, can be effective.

Sometimes negative symptoms are prominent from the first. For other people with schizophrenia, positive/psychotic symptoms are the most obvious signs of illness, but then they may fade away, leaving only negative symptoms.

Negative symptoms may lead to a decline in a person's ability to converse, and his or her speech may lack inflection and/or content, and the facial expression may become unchanging or 'blank'. People with negative symptoms may be inattentive to their surroundings and to the needs and emotions of others, and this can be misinterpreted by family members who see the person as uncaring, hurtful and callous.

Negative symptoms may lead to a lack of energy and initiative, a reduced interest in things going on socially, and recreational activities and social relationships dwindle away. These negative symptoms (particularly the lack of get up and go) can be misinterpreted as 'laziness'.

my experience

Dan was the only child of a 'hippy' mother who adopted an alternative lifestyle. They never lived anywhere together for very long, and once he reached school-age, Dan was left for long periods with his grandparents, who provided stability in his life. As Dan grew up, his mother's visits became less and less frequent.

Dan was a popular and intelligent boy at school, and a member of the 'in' crowd. When he was 15 he started using cannabis with his group of friends and he spent a lot of time drinking and partying. He left school with some qualifications, at the age of 16, and then started on a training scheme in motor mechanics. His grandparents remembered him as a cheerful, canny, adolescent who liked motorbikes.

Gradually, Dan started to miss more and more days at work. He would often stay in bed all day. When his grandparents tried to get him up, he would become irritable and aggressive. He lost his job after six months and, as time passed, he stopped going out and would even refuse to see his friends when they called. Dan would often sit for long periods staring into space, smoking cigarettes, and he stopped washing or changing his clothes.

For a long time, Dan's grandparents thought he was 'going through a phase' and that he was becoming 'the same as his mother'. They finally became really worried, and approached the GP. Dan refused to go to the GP surgery and they had a lot of difficulty getting the GP to agree to visit the house. The GP initially felt that Dan was a normal young man, perhaps reacting in some way to his mother's rejection of him, but the GP eventually (and reluctantly) referred Dan to the local Community Mental Health Team, where a diagnosis of schizophrenia was made. This was some four years after the first signs of Dan's altered behaviour. Dan was treated with medication and eventually accommodated in a hostel for the mentally ill, where a daily programme was set up to increase his socialization and improve his daily living skills. Dan was able to return to some supported vocational training, but he has never been able to live independently.

Dan's story illustrates the difficulty of diagnosing schizophrenia when negative symptoms are the main problem. GPs often have no specialist training in psychiatry and may also be reluctant to diagnose schizophrenia because of the **stigma** of that diagnosis, and the perception that the outlook is always poor. However, it is increasingly recognized that early diagnosis and treatment are important for a good outcome, and that treatment has the most impact during the first five years of the illness. In Dan's case, the most important sign that something was wrong, was his rejection of his friends, and his increasing social isolation. A key factor is often the reaction of a young person's friends. Do they feel that there is something strange or weird going on? Most **psychiatrists** would feel that Dan's use of **cannabis** at an early age was the most important risk factor for him developing the illness (see more in Chapter 3).

stigma
Unreasonable and unjustified prejudice within society, caused by ignorance and fear.

psychiatrist
A medically qualified doctor who, following training, specializes in the treatment of mental illness and abnormal behaviour.

cannabis
Illegal street drug. Using cannabis in early adolescence can lead to a four-fold increase in risk of developing schizophrenia.

Cognitive impairment

Even after the positive symptoms of schizophrenia are successfully treated, people report problems with memory and attention. Particular difficulties are associated with verbal memory, attention, vigilance and speed of cognition, and 'executive' abilities, such as planning or organizing, or doing more than one thing at once. People can lose life and social skills and be unable to work.

There is some evidence from large population studies, that, on average, people who are *going* to get schizophrenia may already have a slightly lower Intelligence Quotient (IQ), particularly in the areas of language and planning. Of course, this is an average finding, and there are many people whose intelligence is exceptional, before they become ill. Once schizophrenia has developed the problem is more pronounced, but again cognitive decline is a finding based on averages; there are many individuals whose cognitive functions are completely unimpaired.

Research studies suggest that cognitive problems are not simply a result of medication. Indeed, the problem is worse if the illness is left untreated during the first five years after onset. Studies have shown that treatment with some **antipsychotic medication** can provide protection against loss of cognitive ability, and in some people there may even be improvement. Cognitive impairment does not appear to be correlated to the length of time the person has been ill, or to the presence of psychotic/positive symptoms, or even negative symptoms, but may occur in anyone with schizophrenia.

antipsychotic medication
Drugs used to treat psychosis divided into typicals (older drugs) and atypicals (more recent drugs with a different side-effect profile).

Cognitive impairment in schizophrenia is very important, because it appears to be directly related to social deficits and functional outcome.

Insight

Psychiatrists consider that **insight** is one of the most important predictors of recovery. 'Having insight' means that the person knows that they are ill, and that his/her symptoms are a product of that illness. If someone has insight, they are more likely to accept treatment and to form a positive alliance with their therapist.

insight (of mental illness)
Refers to an individual's capacity to recognize that he/she is mentally unwell.

Who gets schizophrenia and when do they get it?

Anyone can get schizophrenia – any race or social class, no matter how intelligent or successful they are. Everyone, from every walk of life, every age, and every race and nationality is at risk. Even though there is a raised risk of getting the disorder if there has been a family member with the illness, most individuals with schizophrenia are the only person with the illness in their family.

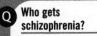

Q Who gets schizophrenia?

A Absolutely anyone can get schizophrenia – male or female young or old and from any walk of life.

Roughly one per cent of the world's population is affected with schizophrenia, which typically comes on in early adulthood, at the time that the brain reaches maturity. However, it can occur at any age, although schizophrenia before puberty is extremely rare.

You may not realize how many people suffer with significant depression or anxiety, as well as the one per cent with schizophrenia. Few people feel able to be open about mental health problems, so if you have not suffered yourself, or seen a close family member suffer, you may know little about it. The box below illustrates the rate of schizophrenia in the population, as well as other mental illnesses.

information

The extent of all mental health problems in the community

Depression	15%
Anxiety	10%
Substance misuse	5%
Bipolar disorder (manic depression)	1%
Schizophrenia	1%

(NB The depression and anxiety in the box are conditions which are *clinically significant and require treatment* – not just everyday moods or worries).

manic depression
An older term for bipolar disorder, though still used.

clinical
Often used in psychiatry to mean 'psychiatrically significant' – hence 'clinical depression', which means depression which needs medical attention as distinct from the everyday 'blues'.

Risk factors for schizophrenia

There is a range of risk factors known to influence the onset of schizophrenia, including adverse events in life, social isolation, or recreational drugs such as cannabis, LSD, amphetamines and cocaine. These and other factors are explored in Chapter 3.

Problems and complications

Depression, suicide and schizophrenia

Although depression and schizophrenia are two entirely separate conditions, people with schizophrenia are particularly likely to become depressed, and this can occur at the beginning of the illness, or later on when it is more established. Depression is an added burden, but it is one that can be relatively easily lifted, because we have effective treatments for depression. Overall, 70 per cent of people with a diagnosis of schizophrenia, will have an episode of depression at some point in the course of their illness. It is very important that depressive symptoms are looked for and treated because depression can make schizophrenia worse and can, in extreme cases, lead to suicide.

Depressive symptoms classically include sad or depressed mood, or loss of interest and pleasure in life. The person may have feelings of emptiness, and may be tearful or irritable. Interest or pleasure in life diminishes, there is poor appetite and weight loss (although sometimes the opposite) and sleep disturbance (either insomnia or the opposite, excessive sleepiness). A depressed person may appear agitated and distressed, may report fatigue or loss of energy, and may have feelings of worthlessness or guilt. In some people with depression there is a diminished ability to think or concentrate, or indecisiveness. Recurrent thoughts of death or suicide often occur. It is important for a doctor to ask about suicide, because people are usually quite frank about their feelings, and asking about suicide is not going to make a suicide attempt more likely.

If you look at the symptoms of depression given above, you can see that there is an overlap with the negative symptoms of schizophrenia, such as withdrawal, or lack of motivation and interest. A separate diagnosis of depression should be suspected if there is a fairly rapid change in the person, or if sadness, tearfulness and suicidal thinking develop. It is an important diagnosis to make, because there are separate treatments for depression and it is usually relatively easily treated.

Depression, suicide and schizophrenia

Seventy per cent of people with a diagnosis of schizophrenia will have an episode of depression, 40 per cent will attempt suicide, and 10 per cent will commit suicide.

Suicide is a problem in the general population, not only for people with schizophrenia, particularly in certain risk groups, such as young men and the unemployed. For people with schizophrenia, men are more likely to commit suicide than women, as are people living alone or living away from their families and people who have suffered recent losses. The loss may be loss of a loved one, but could also be loss of academic achievement or independence. However, the most important factor associated with suicide in people with schizophrenia is depression. There are particular symptoms, such as feelings of worthlessness and/or hopelessness which are most closely associated with suicide.

myth

People with schizophrenia are likely to be violent and homicidal and murder strangers in the street.

fact

This is a very rare situation. Only five per cent of murders are perpetrated by people with psychosis and the number is not rising, contrary to what you may think by the way the media portray people with schizophrenia. Less than one per cent of homicides occur in a situation where a stranger is killed by a mentally ill person. Drug crime and domestic violence account for overwhelmingly more violence in society.

Violence and schizophrenia

There is a widely held belief that people with schizophrenia are likely to be violent and even homicidal. It is certainly the case that someone with acute, untreated psychosis who has threatening and frightening delusions is at risk of becoming violent, but this is uncommon and violence is overwhelmingly restricted to individuals who are extremely unwell and who are usually contained in hospital at the time. There is also a widely held belief that people with schizophrenia are likely to murder strangers on the street. In fact, murders perpetrated by people with schizophrenia are rare, but when they do occur, the media takes notice. In the general population as a whole, homicides are increasing year on year, but homicides by people with schizophrenia remain constant and therefore comprise a diminishing proportion of what is a national problem. A number of violent crimes are drug-related, and there is of course a link between use of drugs and psychosis. However, only about five per cent of homicides are by people who have symptoms of psychosis at the time. Less than one per cent of homicides are in a situation where a stranger is killed by a mentally ill person. There are far more murders by people who are depressed than those who have schizophrenia.

Outcome in schizophrenia

People with schizophrenia typically recover from a first episode of psychotic illness, usually within a number of months. However, until quite recently, the long-term outlook for someone diagnosed with schizophrenia was worrying. While up to 30 per cent of individuals may have a lasting recovery or remission, and another 20 per cent may have substantial improvement, around 50 per cent of people diagnosed with schizophrenia have a chronic long-term illness (sometimes relatively mild, sometimes more severe), which may be episodic or constant in nature.

Looked at another way, the figures drawn from outcome studies of people who became unwell in the 1970s and 1980s show that 60–70 per cent of people with the illness will have some social problems in their lives, often difficulties with occupation or social relationships. However, the general trend from more recent studies is improved. This might be because of new understanding about how to improve the quality of life for people with schizophrenia, or because of the availability of better treatments, or recognition of the importance of optimizing care at an early stage in the illness.

There are a few factors which can help predict whether someone is going to do well after an episode of schizophrenia. The way the illness begins is important. A slow gradual onset is more worrying in terms of long-term outcome than an acute illness. People who are well adjusted in life before they become ill, generally do better. The older the age at onset, the less severe the illness is likely to be. Women tend to do better than men; schizophrenia is generally seen slightly less often and is less severe in women. Women also tend to develop the illness slightly later in life. There are intriguing suggestions that this may be due to the influence of the hormone oestrogen, but this is far from established.

There is a final factor which we can do something about, and that is the 'duration of untreated psychosis'. In other words, it appears that the longer it takes to get effective treatment, the worse the outcome is likely to be.

After the initial episode, many people require long-term medication to remain well, and stopping medication is strongly associated with **relapse**. Of course, it is difficult to remain on medication for years, or even life-long, but improvements in the medication itself, and psychotherapies designed to help people with issues surrounding medication, can help in managing this.

relapse
Re-emergence of illness. Relapse in schizophrenia can be minimized with appropriate medication. It is important to continue with medication even after symptoms have subsided.

Conclusions

Important points to remember

✧ Schizophrenia is a common illness affecting roughly one in a hundred of us. It can affect anyone, at any time, but typically comes on in early adult life at a time when the brain reaches maturity. It can often become chronic. (Note: chronic schizophrenia need not be severe, some cases of chronic illness are relatively mild.)

✧ The symptoms of schizophrenia fall into two groups; (1) psychotic/positive symptoms and (2) negative symptoms. Psychotic symptoms are associated with changes in the part of the brain which processes our understanding of the outside world, and distinguishes our own generated thoughts from everything else going on around us.

✧ The positive/psychotic symptoms of schizophrenia are much more than just hearing voices. Any of the senses can become distorted.

✧ The negative symptoms of schizophrenia are persistent and often the hardest to bear, because the person loses the 'colour' of his or her personality and becomes socially withdrawn and lacking in motivation.

✧ Some people with schizophrenia suffer a deterioration in their intellectual ability; this is most marked where the illness is left untreated for the first five years.

✧ Depression is often an added burden for those with schizophrenia.

✧ People with mental health problems are more likely to be victims than perpetrators of violences.

2 Diagnosing schizophrenia

Difficulties with diagnosis

Although we know what the typical symptoms of schizophrenia are and research has taken us a long way towards understanding the causes of schizophrenia (see Chapter 3), at the moment the diagnosis rests entirely on a psychiatrist's opinion. There are no blood tests or brain scans which can establish the diagnosis with absolute certainty.

information

There are two 'rule books' for diagnosing mental illness which all psychiatrists have to know about and use. Two of these are in use in the UK, the *ICD-10 Classification of Mental and Behavioural Disorders* (World Health Organization, Geneva 1992) and the American system, the '*DSM-IV-TR*' – *Diagnostic and Statistical Manual of Mental Disorders* (4th Edition Text Revision, 2000).

Psychiatrists make their diagnoses by interviewing the person in detail, usually for an hour or more, asking about their symptoms and their life history. Other information may be used, such as information from someone else who is close to the person, or previous psychiatric notes.

> **forensic psychiatry**
> A branch of psychiatry specializing in patients who have committed criminal offences.

information

Training a psychiatrist

After medical school (five years) and one to two years as a junior doctor in medicine and surgery (the 'house doctor' year) psychiatrists undergo a five to seven year training programme in all aspects of mental disorder as well as their chosen speciality. Current specialities include child and adolescent psychiatry, eating disorders, old age psychiatry, learning disability, neuropsychiatry, liaison psychiatry, **forensic psychiatry** and general adult psychiatry.

> **Delusional disorder (paranoia)**
> Diagnosed when there are few features of schizophrenia, or abnormal mood, but the person has prominent delusions (fixed false beliefs) of a grandiose, jealous, persecutory, somatic (relating to physical symptoms) or erotomanic nature (erotomania refers to being secretly loved by someone who may be important or a celebrity). The person with delusional disorder is often able to function normally in many areas of life.

The doctor *can* be certain in most cases that the illness falls into the wider category of psychiatric disorders called 'psychoses' or 'psychotic illness', so called because these illnesses can lead to 'psychosis' as described in Chapter 1.

Within the category 'psychosis', there are two main illnesses, schizophrenia and manic depression, although a host of other diagnostic terms have been proposed over the years, some of which are variants of schizophrenia, while others are thought to be separate conditions. **Delusional disorder** (paranoia) describes a condition where there are few symptoms of psychosis other than prominent delusions. Nowadays manic depression is known as **bipolar disorder** (referring to the two 'poles' of

bipolar disorder
A mood disorder in which an individual alternates between the two 'poles' of depression and the over-excited state of mania. Also known as bipolar affective disorder and manic depression.

mania
A condition of over-excitement associated with hyperactivity and sleeplessness, and sometimes grandiosity. Colloquially known as 'high' it is the opposite of depression and is one of the two poles that makes up bipolar disorder.

the mood – excessively 'up' mood is manic and down is depressed), or 'bipolar affective disorder'. Mood is sometimes known as 'affect'.

It is important to remember that **mania** and depression do not refer to the ordinary ups and downs in mood that we all get. The mood in bipolar disorder is *abnormally* high, or *abnormally* low, and the change in mood lasts for a long time. In the case of depression, a low mood is not counted unless there are at least two full weeks of continuously and abnormally low mood.

Schizophrenia and bipolar disorder are thought to be different illnesses, although both can lead to psychosis.

Bipolar disorder

In bipolar disorder, the mood is particularly unstable and this is thought to be caused by a genetic problem with the regulation of mood. The person can become unusually depressed or, when the mood goes up, the person becomes manic (elated, irritable or euphoric). There are usually well periods in between, when the mood is normal. These episodes of depression or mania can be of varying degrees of severity, and varying lengths of time. Psychosis can develop at times when the depression or mania is particularly severe. The person then loses contact with reality and can begin to hallucinate.

A person with bipolar disorder often has marked mood swings, even when they are essentially well. Interestingly, bipolar disorder is often associated with high artistic ability or creativity, either in the person with bipolar disorder themselves, or in a family member.

There have been many studies of writers, musicians and artists with bipolar disorder (such as Van Gogh).

When someone with bipolar disorder becomes psychotic, the mental state of that person can appear indistinguishable from schizophrenia. How then does the psychiatrist tell the difference?

The only way to decide whether a person has bipolar disorder or schizophrenia is to collect detailed information about how the illness presented, and the pattern of the illness over time. This information (known as 'taking the psychiatric history') usually comes from the person themselves, but often also from family members, friends or carers. Psychiatrists look at the details of the onset of the illness, whether there were previous mood swings or perhaps a milder episode of depression or mania which has become severe. They find out whether the illness comes in episodes, or has gradually developed over a long time. They look for evidence of the negative symptoms of schizophrenia (see Chapter 1). However, it is often not possible to decide whether the person has schizophrenia or bipolar disorder right away on the first visit, and there may be a **working diagnosis** of 'unspecified psychosis' which is used for a time.

Usually, it becomes clear over a matter of weeks or months what the diagnosis is likely to be. However, uncertainties in diagnosis can also arise because people with schizophrenia are particularly likely to become depressed. Seventy per cent of people with schizophrenia will have a depression at some point in the illness and, if they are seen for the first time by the psychiatrist

Q Which psychiatrists look after people with **A** schizophrenia?

General adult psychiatrists care for the majority of people with schizophrenia, usually as part of a **Community Mental Health Team**. Forensic psychiatrists are trained to manage mentally ill criminal offenders, some of whom may also have schizophrenia. Child and adolescent psychiatrists manage very early onset schizophrenia, and old age psychiatrists manage schizophrenia when it begins after the age of 65.

Community Mental Health Team
Multidisciplinary team which cares for people with serious mental disorder in a defined geographical area.

working diagnosis
A diagnosis which is not fully determined, but the one which forms the basis of treatment.

when they are deeply depressed, it may not be clear which came first, the schizophrenia or the depression. Rarely, schizophrenia may lead to an elated or manic mood and again, the same difficulties apply. Things can be even more complicated because schizophrenia sometimes begins with an episode of depression.

my experience

Jim, Geoff and Michael are identical triplets (that is they are genetically identical – with identical DNA). When they were in their early twenties and still living at home, they each developed a psychotic illness and came under the care of the same hospital, but were cared for by different psychiatric teams. Jim and Michael's illnesses started with them hearing voices, becoming very anxious and withdrawn and refusing to go out or even leave their rooms. They were both diagnosed with schizophrenia. Geoff, the third triplet, worked as a bus conductor. A few months after his brothers fell ill, he began to think that he was a very important person in the bus company and developed what he felt were key ideas about the way the timetables should be run. He had racing thoughts and was euphoric in mood. He was diagnosed with bipolar disorder, manic type.

Since the triplets were genetically identical, it was overwhelmingly likely that they had the same illness, and any differences were due to difficulties in diagnosis. This proved to be the case in the end. After several years, Michael recovered sufficiently to come off his medication. He remained well for a short time and then developed a manic episode very similar to Geoff's. Some time later, the same thing happened to Jim. The case histories of the triplets were published in a psychiatric journal to illustrate the difficulties of diagnosis.

Unfortunately, in a proportion of cases (perhaps up to a quarter of people with psychosis) the diagnosis never becomes really clear. There appear to be problems with mood as well as the typical features of schizophrenia discussed in Chapter 1. There is a third psychosis,

schizoaffective disorder, which can be diagnosed in this situation. The symptoms of schizoaffective disorder can be regarded as a mixture between the symptoms of bipolar disorder and schizophrenia, and this diagnosis is sometimes regarded as a 'fudge', made only when the psychiatrist is unsure.

schizoaff...
disorder
A disorder in whic...
mixture of
schizophrenia and
affective (mood)
symptoms are
displayed. There is a
debate in psychiatry as
to whether this is really
a separate disorder.

Changes in diagnosis

There are often changes in diagnosis during the course of someone's illness. The same person may be diagnosed with schizophrenia, bipolar disorder, or schizoaffective disorder at different points in time. About 25 per cent of psychotic patients will have a diagnostic change at some point in their illness. Sometimes this is because the illness itself changes over time, and the correct diagnosis becomes clearer. Sometimes different psychiatrists will have different opinions about the correct diagnosis – remember there are no tests for establishing a correct diagnosis.

Psychiatrists themselves are quite used to, and prepared for, these diagnostic changes. However, they often forget to explain them sufficiently to their patients, who can become very unsettled and lose confidence. Many people think that a diagnosis of bipolar disorder is somehow a 'better' one to have than schizophrenia, perhaps because of the link with creativity, and perhaps because the diagnosis is less feared and less stigmatized (see Chapter 6).

Does a change in diagnosis between psychotic illnesses matter?

Fortunately, diagnostic change is not as important as you might think. Treatment, particularly medication, is targeted to the *symptoms* of the psychotic illnesses – so antipsychotics are used for psychosis, mood stabilizers for instability of mood, and antidepressants for depression. This holds good whatever the underlying diagnosis is felt to be. Interestingly, some of the modern antipsychotic medications (such as olanzapine) are found to be good as mood stabilizers as well as being antipsychotic.

my experience

Joan developed a psychotic illness when she was only 15 years old. She came from a very disturbed family and had spent several years in care. Her illness appeared initially to be typical for schizophrenia, with a gradual onset, social withdrawal, delusions about her family and auditory hallucinations. Joan was admitted to an adolescent unit and treated for and diagnosed with schizophrenia. She made a good recovery, and went on to attempt a career in nursing, but was not successful. Joan became ill again, but this time with an apparently manic episode. She was admitted to an adult psychiatric hospital, where she was diagnosed with bipolar disorder and made a quick recovery. Her new psychiatrist told her that the diagnosis of schizophrenia had been 'wrong'.

Joan reacted very badly to the change in diagnosis. She felt her career problems were due to the diagnosis of schizophrenia and she felt the psychiatrists on the adolescent unit had been negligent, and she should sue them. Her case was taken on by a firm of solicitors, but soon afterwards she was admitted to hospital again, and on this occasion she was diagnosed with schizoaffective disorder. Her legal team felt she no longer had a case and it was dropped. However, Joan never accepted the diagnosis of schizoaffective disorder and continues to believe that her life has been 'blighted' by this 'mistake' of diagnosis.

Confusion about the name 'schizophrenia'

There are older names for the illness, but schizophrenia has stuck. People often say that schizophrenia is an ugly and stigmatizing word and should be changed, but is unlikely that simply changing the name would help to change our perception and understanding about the illness. However, the word itself has caused confusion in its own right.

The actual word 'schizophrenia' is of fairly recent origin; it was coined by the psychiatrist Bleuler in the early twentieth century, to reflect what he saw back then as the cause of schizophrenia. Bleuler thought the brain ('*phrenos*' in Greek) was functionally broken or 'split' (schiz-, which has the same Greek root as 'schism'). Bleuler did *not* mean 'split into two' but rather 'shattered' or 'broken', to reflect his belief that the functions of the brain were no longer coordinated together. In fact Bleuler's ideas about the cause of schizophrenia might well be spot on, but common usage of the term schizophrenia as in 'schizophrenic thinking' is often taken to mean 'two-sided thinking', or 'split brain' and this can lead to confusion with 'split personality'. However, schizophrenia is totally distinct from personality disorder. I once visited a school where a well-meaning teacher wrote a play for her class, in which twins were cast representing two sides of the split personality in schizophrenia. This common view is entirely wrong and unhelpful.

> **myth**
> Schizophrenia is another word for 'split personality'.

> **fact**
> Schizophrenia does *not* mean 'split personality' nor does it have anything to do with multiple (or any other) personality disorder.

Confusion of schizophrenia with personality disorder

personality disorder
Characterized by inflexible and enduring behaviour patterns that impair social functioning. Some borderline disorders can have similarities to schizophrenia.

Some psychiatrists avoid making personality disorder diagnoses as they see them as moral judgements rather than psychiatric problems.

Personality disorder is much more difficult to diagnose than psychosis, and a small number of psychiatrists feel that personality disorders should never be diagnosed, as they are not used to describe an 'illness' but instead describe behavioural traits. The difference between being diagnosed with a personality disorder or with schizophrenia can have enormous significance, as personality disorders are not considered treatable, and a person switched from a diagnosis of schizophrenia to one of personality disorder may lose appropriate treatment and benefits.

The diagnosis of personality disorder can be much harder to make than a psychotic illness. There is no automatic right to treatment or benefits as a personality disorder is not considered an illness.

Our personalities are formed as we grow up, probably as a result of a mixture of genetic factors together with influences on our emotional development during childhood. There is of course an infinite variety of personality, leading to each unique person, but most psychiatrists agree that there are several broad traits in normal people such as neuroticism, extraversion, aggressivity, impulsivity, conscientiousness or reliability and creativity (or intellectual curiosity), and it is the mixture of these traits that define who we are.

Personality traits cross the boundary into 'personality disorder' when they are 'exaggerated, maladaptive, inflexible and cause the person distress', or if they impair the person's ability to function at work or home. Clearly, the boundary is often arbitrary and somewhat speculative, and making a diagnosis of a personality disorder can sometimes indicate little more than social disapproval or a moral judgement.

The distinction between personality disorder and a psychiatric diagnosis is particularly important. While a diagnosis of schizophrenia leads to certain expectations and rights, in terms of care from mental health services or financial benefits, personality disorders do not carry those rights as they are not seen as illnesses. However, the diagnosis of personality disorders, schizophrenia and bipolar disorder are a matter of a psychiatrist's opinion. Sometimes, there is the suspicion that particularly difficult patients are 're-diagnosed' as having a personality disorder rather than schizophrenia so that the local mental health teams do not have to get involved.

To make matters more confusing, individuals with personality disorders tend to develop mental illnesses more frequently than other people. Mentally ill offenders will often have both a personality disorder and a psychotic illness.

Different kinds of personality disorder

This is a complex area. Personality disorders are organized into three **clusters**, known as A, B and C. There are three Cluster A personality disorders:

✧ paranoid
✧ schizoid
✧ schizotypal.

Paranoid personality disorder refers to individuals who are suspiciousness, have a mistrust of others and who are hypersensitive to criticism. **Schizoid personality disorder** is

clusters
Personality disorders are arranged into three clusters: A (paranoid, schizoid, schizotypal); B (antisocial, borderline, historic, narcissistic); C (avoidant, dependent, obsessive-compulsive). There is often considerable overlap within each cluster.

where a person shows discomfort in social interactions and has extreme introversion. **Schizotypal personality disorder** is the most controversial and difficult to explain of all the personality disorders but basically refers to a solitary, underachieving, hypersensitive character who has rather odd preoccupations, as well as unusual thinking and speech. A proportion of people with schizoid and schizotypal personality disorders go on to get schizophrenia.

The overlap of cluster 'A' personality disorders with schizophrenia can be particularly problematic where schizophrenia develops gradually in a young person who becomes more and more odd and withdrawn. Many psychiatrists consider that, with this presentation, a trial of antipsychotic medication is worthwhile, whatever the diagnosis ultimately proves to be.

my experience

Jeremy had always been a withdrawn, isolated child. He was tall and clumsy and very bad at sport. His overwhelming interest in life was the *Star Trek* TV and film series and, as a teenager, he taught himself Klingon (a made-up language associated with the series) and collected all the *Star Trek* episodes. Jeremy did quite well in his GCSEs, and went on to college, where he got 'A' levels in maths and economics (although the grades were low). As far as his parents knew, he never made any friends apart from one other 'Trekkie'. He spent all his free time at home, where his friend would visit once or twice a week. After college he made some attempt to get a job, but never managed to get one. When he was 20, his parents moved house, and Jeremy lost contact with his 'Trekkie' friend, and became even more isolated and withdrawn and spent all day in his bedroom. His interest in *Star Trek* seemed to fade. Finally his parents asked for him to be seen by a psychiatrist.

At the clinic, Jeremy was aloof, withdrawn and said very little. He denied any problems with his mood or any psychotic symptoms at all. He was unable to say how he spent his time and appeared to have very little to say on any topic. Depression was suspected and Jeremy was given an antidepressant but after two months this had made no difference, and Jeremy was then started on one of the atypical antipsychotics as well as the antidepressant. After a further six months Jeremy's parents reported a gradual improvement in his sociability. His dad helped him to get a job in the local supermarket and Jeremy has held this job down and socializes with the family, although with no one else. He continues to attend the psychiatric clinic on a six-monthly basis; no diagnosis (apart from schizoid personality disorder) has ever been made.

There are four cluster B personality disorders:

- ✧ histrionic
- ✧ narcissistic
- ✧ antisocial
- ✧ borderline.

Histrionic personality disorder is loosely defined, but refers to individuals who are dramatic, attention-seeking and demanding. **Narcissistic personality disorder** is diagnosed in individuals who have an exaggerated sense of self-importance, together with a lack of regard for others and a craving for admiration and gratification. The best known cluster B personality disorder is **antisocial personality disorder** (also known as psychopathy or sociopathy). Such individuals can be charming, unreliable, manipulative, lack remorse and are particularly likely to engage in criminal activity or drug abuse. (Antisocial in this context does not mean 'bolshie' but is used in a much stronger sense, meaning persistently against society.)

my experience

Andrew was a difficult and demanding child. His parents divorced when he was only five, and he had a very poor relationship with his stepfather who abused him physically and sexually from a young age. Andrew never settled to anything at school, and he engaged in petty crime and heavy drug abuse when he was an adolescent. When he was arrested for severely beating up his girlfriend, Andrew reacted by overdosing on paracetamol. He then came under the care of the local mental health team, and was admitted to hospital where he reported hearing the voice of an older man telling him to kill himself. Andrew was diagnosed schizophrenic and he was tried on a variety of antipsychotic medications, without any effect.

Andrew's behaviour in hospital continued to be very difficult. He would smoke cannabis and drink on the ward, take the belongings of other patients, and he was also suspected of raping a female patient, although this could not be proved. Andrew's behaviour was felt to be deliberate and intentional. The diagnosis was changed to that of antisocial personality disorder with borderline features, and Andrew was discharged quite quickly and was not offered follow-up. Andrew's mother was distraught.

After discharge, Andrew started to sleep rough. He continued to meet patients from the ward in the hospital grounds, supplying them with cannabis and taking money from the most vulnerable. As time passed, Andrew's behaviour became more and more disorganized, and he was increasingly violent and aggressive, but the local mental health team refused to see him and said he should be dealt with by the police.

After a break-in at the local off-licence, Andrew was placed on remand, where he was seen by a forensic psychiatrist. Andrew was felt to have treatment resistant schizophrenia as well as an antisocial personality disorder and he was committed to a secure hospital where he remains to date, although he has made some response to treatment.

Andrew's mother remains convinced that he had a diagnosis of schizophrenia all along, and that the decision of the local mental health team to discharge him without follow-up was responsible for many of Andrew's subsequent difficulties and his eventual placement in a secure hospital.

The fourth personality disorder in cluster B, **borderline personality disorder**, has become a controversial diagnosis, with considerable confusion with psychotic illnesses, both schizophrenia and bipolar disorder. It is thought that in some people borderline personality disorder develops when there is an interaction between a genetic vulnerability to stress or problems with the regulation of mood, together with some kind of emotional trauma during childhood. For example, people who have an anxious disposition, and who also suffered emotional trauma in childhood from abuse or neglect, may develop chronic fear of abandonment, impulsivity and instability of mood. They may be manipulative, demanding and self-serving, and they may self-mutilate or harm themselves in other ways, such as overdosing on medication. They may have problems with alcohol and illegal drugs. People with borderline personality disorder may also report psychotic experiences.

Multiple personality disorder is thought to be a rare, extreme form of borderline personality disorder. It is thought that these individuals may have suffered a trauma, and that this is so great that their personality literally 'splits' in order to protect the person from excessive emotion. The use of the word 'split' leads to confusion with schizophrenia.

The distinction between borderline personality disorder and schizophrenia often causes diagnostic dilemma. However, individuals with borderline personality disorder tend not to have negative symptoms, cognitive decline or a deteriorating course. Fortunately, individuals with borderline personality disorder do tend to

myth
Antisocial behaviour rules out a diagnosis of schizophrenia and suggests personality disorder.

fact
Some people have both personality disorder and schizophrenia.

respond well to antipsychotic medication, perhaps because the medication stabilizes their mood. Psychotherapy is also very important, but because of the background of emotional difficulties or damage in childhood, and the tendency of these people to become very emotionally dependent, psychotherapy for this condition is difficult and specialized.

my experience

Tammy had an extremely disrupted childhood. She was the oldest of four children, all with different fathers. Tammy's mother would leave the children alone for long periods, with Tammy in charge of the younger ones. Tammy's father was a distant figure in her life, but when she was 11 her mother dumped Tammy with her father, and took the three younger children to France. Tammy described being sexually abused by her mother's boyfriend from the age of nine, and it was after she told her mother about this that she was sent to live with her father. Her father was an alcoholic and was violent when drunk. Tammy's stepmother disliked her. Within six months of moving to her father's house, Tammy was taken into care. She had little contact with either parent for many years after that.

As a teenager, Tammy's behaviour was very difficult. She drank and used drugs and was promiscuous from a young age. She was offered counselling and support but rejected it. Tammy was attractive and outgoing and after leaving care she got a job in a boutique. This was one of many jobs she obtained and quickly lost, sometimes being suspected of stealing from the till, sometimes turning up drunk, and often not turning up at all. Tammy had several relationships with men, one of whom beat her so badly she was admitted to hospital. After this Tammy formed a strong relationship with a psychotherapist, whom she told about her unhappy and abused childhood. Tammy described herself as having several different personalities. One spoke with a French accent, another was 'the inner Tammy' who protected her, and talked to her. Tammy described being able to hear Tammy's voice inside her head whenever she felt alone or stressed. At times, Tammy found herself in a strange man's bed in the morning, and she knew she had been taken over by the personality Jade, who liked sex.

> Tammy's psychotherapist arranged for her to be referred to the local community mental health team (CMHT), who made a diagnosis of borderline personality disorder. Tammy was not prescribed medication, but was offered further psychotherapy, which she refused, preferring to stay with her original therapist. Sadly, only a few weeks after being seen by the CMHT Tammy was found dead with high levels of alcohol and cocaine in her bloodstream. It could not be established whether the overdose was accidental or deliberate.

The final cluster of personality disorders is C, which includes:

✧ obsessive compulsive personality disorder (characterized by inflexible perfectionism and a wish to control)
✧ avoidant personality disorder (characterized by low self-esteem, social awkwardness and a fear of being viewed negatively by others)
✧ dependent personality disorder (where individuals are excessively 'clinging', fear separation and have desire to be taken care of).

These problems can be seen as exaggerations of neurotic, obsessional or anxious traits, and there is little diagnostic confusion with schizophrenia.

Confusion of schizophrenia with drug-induced psychosis

A number of drugs are known to cause psychosis directly. Drugs that alter perception and mood, without causing disorientation, are known as 'hallucinogenic' drugs – because they cause hallucinations. There are many such drugs, but the most commonly known are amphetamine, cannabis, cocaine, ecstasy, ketamine, LSD, mescaline, phencyclidine (angel dust), psilocybin and psilocin (magic mushrooms). Alcohol can also cause psychosis in some cases, as can anabolic steroids.

Hallucinogens can cause acute anxiety and panic ('bad trips'), persisting flashbacks and prolonged psychosis. A true drug-induced psychosis can be recognized because it arises during a period of intoxication with the drug, which can be confirmed by a positive drug screen in blood or urine and, most importantly, there is resolution of the psychosis as soon as the individual stops using the drug.

However, there are many cases where the distinction between drug-induced psychosis and schizophrenia is very unclear. A period of substance misuse often precedes the development of typical schizophrenia, and substance misuse is thought to be a strong risk factor for schizophrenia. It is also the case that in people who already have schizophrenia, the use of hallucinogenic drugs can make matters much worse, causing relapse and/or increased severity of the illness.

Once a period of psychosis persists far beyond the period of intoxication with a particular drug, the distinction between schizophrenia and drug-induced psychosis may not be useful or practical. The same antipsychotic drugs are necessary treatments whether or not hallucinogenic drugs were implicated in the onset, and the outcome is generally similar, whether or not hallucinogenic drugs were involved at the outset, although persistent drug abusers tend to have more difficult and complicated problems (on account of what is known as **dual diagnosis** – generally taken to refer to a combination of drug-related

dual diagnosis
In psychiatry this refers to substance abuse (usually street drugs and/or alcohol) in addition to a diagnosis of another psychiatric disorder.

problems and psychosis). In general, health services aimed at people with drug problems (substance misuse) will not be geared up to dealing with individuals who are using drugs and have become psychotic.

Even where there is a clear-cut drug induced psychosis, which gets better once the drug is stopped, a high proportion (perhaps 50 per cent) of patients will have further episodes of psychosis even if they never use that drug again. In these cases the drug has triggered a separate psychotic illness.

Some families find it comforting and less stigmatizing to characterize the illness in their loved one as drug-induced psychosis rather than schizophrenia, but it is important to remember that, in practical terms, there may be little difference. Dan's story, in Chapter 8, illustrates a cannabis-related psychosis.

Subtypes of schizophrenia

Sometimes, a diagnosis of schizophrenia is qualified by a **subtype**. You may see a diagnostic subtype applied to a particular case, so it is helpful to describe them. These subtypes are descriptive, and are *not particularly important* in terms of outcome, treatment or research, because they are defined by the symptoms the person has at the time of evaluation, and may change over time. Often a person may show symptoms of more than one subtype.

Standard diagnostic criteria used by psychiatrists (see Chapter 2) list four subtypes of schizophrenia:

subtype
The subtypes of schizophrenia are paranoid, disorganized or hebephrenic, catatonic and residual. These terms are used less and less and have little bearing on outcome or treatment. The diagnosis of schizophrenia is much more significant than the precise subtype.

✧ paranoid
✧ disorganized or hebephrenic

✧ catatonic
✧ residual.

These are not important in terms of outcome or treatment.

Paranoid schizophrenia is diagnosed when the individual has relatively prominent delusions or hallucinations with well-preserved cognitive functioning and presentation. There is a tendency for the delusions to have persecutory or grandiose themes. The onset of the illness is generally later than other forms of schizophrenia, and the outlook may be better. This condition generally responds well to antipsychotic drugs. It is sometimes wrongly thought that this is the worst kind of schizophrenia and that everyone with this diagnosis is always a danger to others.

Disorganized or **hebephrenic schizophrenia** is a particularly severe form where the person's behaviour appears disorganized, inappropriate and empty of purpose. There may be odd mannerisms or grimaces, senseless laughter and delusions and speech is often rambling and incoherent, with the 'thought disorder' described above. Negative symptoms appear early on in the illness.

Catatonic schizophrenia is rarely seen in industrialized countries, for reasons which are poorly understood. It is a very unusual presentation, with strange peculiarities of movement and behaviour, for example extreme immobility with a resistance to being moved, inappropriate posturing, mutism, or repeating the last thing said by the examiner.

The term **residual schizophrenia** is used when the individual has had one characteristic episode of schizophrenia, but there are no longer prominent positive symptoms, and the negative symptoms dominate the picture.

There is a further subtype which is seldom used: 'simple' schizophrenia. This refers to a condition where there is a slow development of negative symptoms, with a progressive decline in social performance and increasing lack of initiative and motivation, but without any positive symptoms being seen.

Conclusions

✧ The most important decision for a doctor to make is whether the person is psychotic or not. A decision between the various diagnoses *within* the category of psychosis may take longer, and is not important in terms of immediate treatment.

✧ There is some overlap between schizophrenia and some personality disorders.

✧ The diagnostic decision between a psychotic illness and a personality disorder can make the difference between getting appropriate treatment and benefits or getting nothing at all.

✧ Illegal drugs can lead to drug-induced psychosis. Although this is a separate diagnosis to schizophrenia, drug-induced progresses to schizophrenia in a large number of cases.

✧ Those with 'dual-diagnosis' (schizophrenia and drug abuse) are particularly difficult to treat as specialist services may not be available.

3 Current research in schizophrenia

Risk factors for schizophrenia include the following:

✧ genetic susceptibility
✧ drug abuse (particularly at a young age)
✧ prenatal or birth complications
✧ seasonal variation of birth
✧ immigration status and ethnicity
✧ urban birth and upbringing
✧ social isolation/adverse events
✧ slightly higher rates in males.

Genetic research

Early researchers considered the cause of schizophrenia to be genetic, with genes involved in a simple 'cause and effect' fashion. They did not realize that schizophrenia, like other common illnesses which affect the population such as heart disease, diabetes or high blood pressure, is genetic to some extent, but the situation is much more complicated than that. Fully genetic conditions such as haemophilia, cystic fibrosis or Huntington's Chorea are comparatively rare, and their straightforward patterns of inheritance (known as 'Mendelian' inheritance patterns because they are similar to those Mendel found in his peas) are easy to demonstrate. In contrast, schizophrenia is inherited more like heart disease – there appears to be some tendency for the illness to cluster in certain families, but it does not correspond to straightforward genetic patterns, and other risk factors must be involved.

Although schizophrenia is not caused by a single gene, genes remain very influential. There have been several major, long-term studies in large populations which have shown that schizophrenia is definitely inherited to some extent. The Danish adoption studies are a good example. In Denmark there are good national statistics, so the lifetime outcome of various groups of children can be discovered. By comparing the rate of schizophrenia occurring in adopted children who have a biological parent with schizophrenia, but are brought up by a different family, to adopted children with no schizophrenia in their biological parents, it can be shown that having a biological parent with schizophrenia confers a risk of developing the illness of about ten times that in the general population. The rate is the same in children who are not adopted at all, but are brought up by a biological parent with schizophrenia. Where both parents have schizophrenia, the risk for the child is much higher and approaches 50 per cent. By way of contrast, adopted children with no schizophrenia in their biological parents, who happen to be brought up by an adoptive parent who has developed schizophrenia, do not have a

> **myth**
> Schizophrenia has a simple genetic cause, such as a single faulty gene, and this gene could be eliminated from the population if the people carrying it were identified and did not pass the gene on to their children.

> **fact**
> There will never be a simple 'cause and effect' between any given gene and schizophrenia. Genes are likely to confer a *susceptibility* to develop schizophrenia, so many people will possess one or many of these genes and stay well their entire lives.

raised risk. Overall, the evidence from these studies shows that genes account for about 80 per cent of the cause (known as **heritability**) of schizophrenia. This 80 per cent heritability is a statistical figure for the population as a whole. We don't know what the heritability is for any particular individual; some people may have a more genetically influenced illness than others.

heritability
The degree to which a disorder is inherited.

Nowadays, we are not looking for single 'simple cause and effect' genes, but instead for those genes that confer **susceptibility**. This means that possessing one or more of these genes would make it more likely that you would get schizophrenia – but would by no means make it certain. We expect that susceptibility genes also exist for other common illnesses, such as heart disease. The concept of susceptibility is easily understood if you think of something like fair skin and the risk of skin cancer. People with fair skin have a raised risk of skin cancer. Skin colour is genetic, so the genes for fair skin are associated with skin cancer, but another risk factor, exposure to the sun, is also necessary for the cancer to occur.

susceptibility
In gentetics, having a raised risk on account of genetic make-up. In schizophrenia this does not mean that a person will inevitably get the disorder.

There are projects underway in the UK, Europe and America to screen whole populations, looking for regions of the genetic code, or variations of known genes, which may confer susceptibility for various illnesses. Once these are found, there will need to be further projects to find out exactly what this susceptibility means and what other risk factors may be involved.

It seems likely that there are a variety of susceptibility genes involved for schizophrenia, each of comparatively weak effect. Some likely genes have already been identified, but exactly how they confer susceptibility is unknown. The genes are thought to interact with each other and also with other non-genetic factors affecting the person from development in the womb onwards. These 'non-genetic' factors might be something affecting the early development of the baby in the womb – perhaps to do with the health of the mother. They might be to do with social stresses affecting the person in childhood or later on, or they might be to do with drugs, used later in life, such as cannabis, amphetamines or cocaine. The susceptibility genes could act in a variety of ways; for example, they could cause the brain cells in the foetus to develop in ways which make it easier for psychosis to develop. These genes could also influence the way the brain matures throughout childhood, or they could interact with a third factor, such as hallucinogenic drugs. So far, there are no certain answers, and while there are some promising leads, the genetic basis of schizophrenia is going to take some time to unravel.

my experience

Jenny's experience: Both Jenny's brothers developed schizophrenia when they were in their late teens and an uncle also had the illness. There were rumours that more distant male relatives may also have had mental illness. Jenny had a difficult childhood on account of her brother's problems, and she grew up believing her grandmother, who said there was a genetic problem affecting the boys in the family. When she got married, Jenny actually considered having a termination if she became pregnant with a son, because she felt her sons would be at high risk for schizophrenia. When she was told a termination would never be sanctioned on such grounds, Jenny was afraid to have children at all. Jenny nearly missed out on having a family because she had this misunderstanding about genes and schizophrenia. Jenny did not consider that the heavy drug use of both her brothers was likely to have been implicated in their illnesses, and she did not know that there is no evidence at all for schizophrenia following the male (or female) line in a particular family.

myth

Schizophrenia affects exclusively males (or females) in any given family.

fact

The appearance of schizophrenia in males or females in any family is purely random. There is no association of schizophrenia with the sex chromosome.

Using brain scans to understand schizophrenia

There was great excitement when modern brain scanners, introduced in the 1970s, showed that some people with schizophrenia had clearly observable anatomical abnormalities in the brain, which were present from early on in the illness.

The excitement was short-lived, however, because no abnormalities have been found which are *specific* to schizophrenia. In every case, there are many people who are entirely well, who also have one of these abnormalities in the brain. There are also many people with schizophrenia who have an apparently 'perfect' brain. The association appears to be statistical – more people with schizophrenia have such abnormalities than people who do not have schizophrenia.

Overall, studies show that, statistically, parts of the brain, particularly the temporal lobes and the **hippocampus** (part of the limbic system) tend to be decreased in size, and the surrounding fluid spaces are correspondingly enlarged, in schizophrenia.

Researchers looked at reasons why parts of the brain might be smaller in schizophrenia but this does not appear to be the result of some illness process destroying brain cells (which is the case

hippocampus
Part of the brain; thought possibly to be implicated in schizophrenia.

for Alzheimer's dementia, for example). Detailed studies of the actual brain cells themselves are difficult, because of course the person has to be dead for the brain cells to be studied, and reliably diagnosed with schizophrenia before they die. However, there is an emerging understanding that there is a difference in the connections between the brain cells in schizophrenia – the 'wiring' of the brain is different and also that, in some cases, there may be fewer cells in certain areas.

There remains a great deal that is unknown about the brain in schizophrenia. We do not know if there are particular patterns of abnormal 'wiring' which are specific to schizophrenia, or how any abnormal connections in the brain relate to actual symptoms. We do not know when these changes occur; perhaps they develop as the brain forms in the womb. We know that a number of genes are involved, but how they relate to any brain abnormalities remains a mystery.

Using brain scans to understand the symptoms of schizophrenia

Brain scanners that allow us to see the brain actually working can also show us what happens when someone hallucinates.

It has long been thought that hallucinations occur when the processes involved in the brain when you think or speak words to yourself, go wrong in some way. For example, as you read this paragraph, think of a poem or the words of a song. You know that you have thought of the words yourself, but in schizophrenia the brain seems to become 'muddled' between things you think or say to yourself, and things you hear from outside. Similar muddles are thought to account for hallucinations in other senses like sight, touch and smell. In some people suffering from schizophrenia, there are even vibrations in the larynx which correspond to the hallucinations they are hearing, as if they are literally 'talking' their hallucinations, and in some extreme cases, the person thinks they are hallucinating words which they are actually saying out loud.

my experience

Tricia had an extremely stressful time in her mid-fifties. She had an unpleasant divorce, and then took up with a fraudster who took all her money. As a consequence she had to sell her house and lost her job. She moved to a small cottage in an isolated area, where she knew nobody. Soon after she moved, Tricia became unwell, and she began to hear an old lady speaking to her. Tricia believed that the old lady was broadcasting to her from a radio hidden somewhere in the house, telling her that she was going to go bankrupt and be out on the street. She was convinced that this was happening and when her family were doubtful, she was able to produce tape recordings of the voice. Tricia's family recognized the voice as Tricia herself.

Tricia was admitted to hospital. She continued to hear the 'old lady', while staff reported hearing Tricia talking to herself in her room, for hour after hour. With a lot of explanation, and her consent, a video recorder was placed in Tricia's room and it showed her 'speaking' her own hallucinations. Tricia's illness responded to a low dose of medication and her hallucinations stopped. She understood what had happened to her. Part of her aftercare plan ensured that Tricia made links with her local community and started voluntary work. She has remained well and active ever since.

PET

Position emission tomography: brain imaging which can investigate the functioning of the brain three-dimensionally. Entails the injection of drugs which are traceable radioactively.

SPECT

Single photon emission computed tomography. Brain imaging technique which can investigate the functioning of the brain three-dimensionally. Entails the injection of drugs which are traceable radioactively.

The early studies of brain function, in the 1980s, used brain scanners such as **PET** scanners or **SPECT** scanners, which could show only roughly which part of the brain was activated at any given time. They could not provide the detailed picture we see with a present day **MRI** scan, which shows the exact anatomy of the brain. An MRI scanner uses the (tiny) forces in the brain after it has been magnetized to build up a picture of the brain structure and is safe except for people for whom being magnetized might be dangerous (anyone with metal in their brain from a plate or operation). PET and SPECT use radioactivity and so the number of scans a person can have is limited. The principle involved in PET and SPECT is simple; the parts of the brain which are actively working are taking up the most oxygen and glucose. If the research subject is breathing radioactive oxygen, or has been injected with radioactive glucose, then a scanner which can detect radiation will 'see' which part of the brain is most active, at the time. For the first time, we could show which parts of the brain were active when someone was actually hallucinating. Interestingly, with auditory hallucinations the parts of the brain which detect speech were active, but also the regions of the brain concerned with generating language.

More recent research with better scanners has shown the process in more detail, and the results suggest that there is a sequence of brain activity which leads to auditory hallucinations. Subjective memories (rather like your own memories when you thought about that poem earlier) begin the process. But in schizophrenia these memories also trigger the language and speech systems of the brain, perhaps because of some faulty connection. Then another part of the brain lends 'emotional significance' to the process, and finally the auditory cortex, the part of the brain which allows us to hear, is also triggered. There are no answers yet for visual, olfactory or sensory

MRI
Magnetic resonance imaging: a brain imaging technique able to detect variation in brain structure. Safe for patients to be scanned regularly (unless they have pacemakers or metal plates).

Q I have recently been diagnosed with schizophrenia – should I have a brain scan?

A The current answer to this question is 'yes', in case you have one of the conditions in the list below, which may rarely present like schizophrenia, and which would require a fundamentally different form of treatment.

However, in general, brain scans cannot be used to rule in, or rule out, a diagnosis of schizophrenia. The research findings referred to above in relation to schizophrenia are based on statistical groups, and cannot be generalized to individuals.

hallucinations, but most people think these occur in a similar fashion.

A sideline of this research is that psychiatrists are once more becoming interested in the actual content of hallucinations. For many years people with schizophrenia were discouraged from talking about their hallucinations, because the content was thought to be meaningless, but now we understand that they may represent someone's worst fears or worries; it is worth addressing these fears in psychotherapy tailored for psychosis.

The significance of brain scan information for individuals

In most cases, a brain scan is not going to be terribly informative in an individual case, although the process of participating in research can be very reassuring.

my experience

John had been unwell with schizophrenia for nearly 15 years when he agreed to participate in a research project looking at the brains of people who heard voices. John was asked to lie down in the scanner and press a buzzer when he heard a voice. The pictures of his brain when he heard a voice, were compared to the activity in John's brain when he actually heard a researcher talking, and to the activity in his brain when he recited words to himself. Afterwards, the researchers demonstrated the pictures of his brain working, and showed John that the hallucinations corresponded to his own brain generating, and hearing, words. John said that, although the hallucinations remained distressing, he actually felt very comforted by the knowledge that they were generated by his own brain.

However, as many as ten per cent of people with a diagnosis of schizophrenia may have some abnormality in the brain, and sometimes, albeit rarely, this may be something like a brain tumour, or brain injury or infection, which would require a different form of treatment. It is accepted as good practice amongst psychiatrists to scan someone with a first episode of psychosis.

Conditions which can be identified using MRI brain scans include:

✧ strokes
✧ tumours
✧ bleeding into the brain
✧ increased pressure on the brain
✧ injury
✧ epilepsy
✧ multiple sclerosis
✧ certain infections.

What is dopamine and why is it important?

Dopamine is a **neurotransmitter**, which is a chemical involved in making connections within parts of the brain. Some brain cells use dopamine to pass messages to and from each other, in particular the brain cells in areas of the brain associated with psychosis. Since the 1960s, we have known that drugs which release more dopamine in the brain make the psychotic symptoms of schizophrenia worse, while drugs which block it, can improve these psychotic symptoms. Modern brain scanners can show dopamine in action.

One important function of dopamine in the brain is to allow the person to react appropriately to interesting, significant or crisis events. When something important happens, dopamine is released and you pay attention! But research has shown that the brains of people

dopamine
Dopamine is a neurotransmitter and it is thought that overactivity in the dopamine systems is implicated in the generation of psychotic symptoms in schizophrenia. Antipsychotic drugs work, in part, by blocking dopamine.

neurotransmitter
A chemical messenger in the brain.

with schizophrenia release more dopamine than they should at times when there isn't anything much going on, and so the brain gives 'crisis meaning' to ordinary events. If, for example, you release a lot of dopamine when you hear a car passing on the road, then this could seem enormously significant and important, or if you are releasing too much dopamine when you see two people talking, then it can seem that something is going on; perhaps they are conspiring against you. Of course, the person concerned has no idea what is happening in their brain, they just react to what they *perceive* to be going on with anxiety or worry, and they try to make sense of it.

Much of the medication used in schizophrenia (and other psychoses) works by blocking dopamine. This prevents the excess dopamine being released, and so prevents 'crisis meaning' being attributed to non-significant events or situations. One of the side effects of medication, however, can be that the person can no longer respond appropriately to real crises. This is not so much of a problem with some of the newer medication.

Non-genetic risk factors

As noted earlier in the section on genetics, genetic research is not likely to provide a simple answer in the search for the cause of schizophrenia. There are likely to be several genes involved, none of which leads to schizophrenia in a simple 'cause and effect' manner, but instead they confer susceptibility. Whether the person develops schizophrenia or not will also depend on other factors.

Cannabis and other drugs

Drug abuse is one of the most important environmental factors associated with schizophrenia. It has been known for decades that taking amphetamines and cocaine (known as 'hallucinogenic' drugs) can lead to psychosis, and drug abuse with hallucinogenic drugs is a known antecedent to both the first episode of schizophrenia and also causes relapse.

Recently, there has been powerful evidence that cannabis is also associated with schizophrenia, particularly when cannabis is used in the teenage years, before the brain is fully formed. 'Modern' cannabis, for example, skunk can be about seven times as powerful as the cannabis that was used in the 1960s, so perhaps this effect was not so marked in the past.

It has been suggested that the use of cannabis as a teenager could double the risk of developing schizophrenia. The younger the person begins to use cannabis, the greater the risk; using cannabis in early adolescence can lead to a four-fold increase in risk of developing schizophrenia.

Unfortunately, cannabis also has a calming effect so, while it is actually being taken or smoked, it can temporarily alleviate the fear and anxiety caused by the symptoms that it may have helped produce.

Dan's story, which you can find in Chapter 8, is a good illustration of the problems of cannabis and schizophrenia.

Factors associated with birth and childhood development

Influences that are non-genetic come into play as soon as the egg is fertilized. It is known that maternal stress or illness during pregnancy can cause problems for the developing baby, and there is a known association between birth complications and the development of schizophrenia.

People who develop schizophrenia are twice as likely as other people to have suffered problems before, during, or shortly after birth. These are problems affecting the pregnant mother such as ill-health, bleeding during pregnancy, low birth weight or developmental problems in the baby, or problems associated with lack of oxygen around the time of birth. The age of the father is also thought to be a risk factor, with fathers over the age of 50 conferring an increased risk for schizophrenia to their offspring.

Factors affecting the pregnant mother which may confer an increased risk of schizophrenia in the offspring are thought to include prenatal exposure to infections such as influenza, rhesus incompatibility, nutritional deficiency in the first three months, or major stress (such as a death or disaster).

We also know that children who go on to develop schizophrenia later in life are more likely to show problems with language, coordination, emotional development and intelligence than those who do not. Rachel's story (Chapter 6) about her adopted daughter Sara, is a typical history showing these problems.

We have known for a long time that males tend to develop schizophrenia at an earlier age than females. Recent research has also shown that schizophrenia is also slightly more frequent in males. Reasons for this are unknown.

An intriguing, poorly understood risk factor is the association of schizophrenia (and a number of other conditions) with winter/early spring birth.

This has a relatively slight effect, but the association has been shown in many populations (including those in the southern hemisphere), over decades of research. As yet, we have no idea why this should be the case.

Ethnicity and immigration status

Recent large-scale studies have shown that first-generation migrants have a two- to three-fold increased risk of developing schizophrenia, and second generation migrants have an even higher risk. The risk is greater if the migrants come from areas where the majority of the population have a black skin colour. There is *not* the same risk in the country of origin, suggesting that it is something to do with the process of migration. There is increasing evidence that social isolation is also a risk factor for schizophrenia in non-migrant populations.

Most research has focused on adversity in adult life to explain this increased risk. Increased rates of drug abuse, social adversity (e.g. racial discrimination) and social isolation have all been suggested as possible explanations. However, there may be increased risk in the earliest stages of life, or before birth, on account of infections or vitamin deficiencies in pregnant mothers. For example, migrant women with black skin colour, moving from a sunny rural climate to a European city where there is less opportunity for exposure to the sun, may suffer vitamin D deficiency, and vitamin D deficiency in the mother during pregnancy may confer a risk of schizophrenia in the offspring.

The high rate of schizophrenia diagnosed in black immigrant populations cannot simply be due to overdiagnosis caused by institutional racism in mental health services, as some people have suggested. Even though there are more black and ethnic minorities in secure settings, this finding could be due to a delay in some ethnic groups seeking help, which could result in the psychosis being more severe before people from these backgrounds are seen by services. More research is needed to understand this problem.

Urban birth and upbringing

The risk of developing schizophrenia is higher in those people born and brought up in urban environments compared to those born and brought up in the countryside. It is tempting to speculate why this should be the case – life is more difficult in the city, with more infection, drug abuse and exposure to adversity, but we don't know for sure.

Adverse life situations and events

It is not thought that unpleasant life events, such as loss of a loved one, or some other adversity are actually causal in schizophrenia, but such problems are thought to contribute to relapse, and may also start the illness off in someone who is already very vulnerable.

Conclusions

✧ The cause of schizophrenia, in any individual, is likely to be a complicated interaction between a number of weak 'susceptibility' genes together with risk factors in the environment.

✧ Overall, genes account for about 80 per cent of the cause.

✧ The only environmental risk factor that we can realistically do anything about is drug abuse, which is a particularly strong risk factor for those who abuse drugs at a young age.

✧ Many other risk factors are poorly understood but, in general, it is always wise to attend to physical health and wellbeing, particularly in pregnancy.

CHAPTER

4

History, families, myths and stigma

If a young adult develops a serious illness such as schizophrenia, the first reaction of the parents may be to blame themselves for their poor parenting. Modern research evidence shows that family upbringing is very unlikely to be responsible. However, there have, in the past, been theories suggesting exactly the opposite. These old ideas led to powerful and erroneous myths about the illness, and these myths have hung on in some quarters and can still lead to distress today. It is worth taking a little time to understand the history of schizophrenia to see how some of the myths developed and how their legacy has contributed to the stigma·which still surrounds schizophrenia.

Early genetic theories

The early scientists and psychiatrists thought that there might be a single faulty gene which was responsible for causing schizophrenia. Research began in the late-nineteenth century when the psychiatrist, Emil Kraepelin (whom many psychiatrists consider was the father of modern psychiatry), noticed that some cases of schizophrenia appeared to be related to damage to the developing baby in the womb, for example, from alcoholism in the mother, while other cases appeared to be 'hereditary' – that is they ran in families. At the time, the science of genetics was newly discovered and fashionable. In fact, there was no real concept of genetics at all before the middle of the nineteenth century, when Darwin published *On the Origin of Species*, and Gregor Mendel's earlier foundation work on modern genetics using peas was first noticed by the scientific community.

Early scientific enthusiasm for genetics as the key to schizophrenia had a very unfortunate by-product. In the early twentieth century, the term **eugenics** was used to describe the possibility of cleaning up the human gene pool by removing faulty genes. Such ideas were widespread across Europe but, most significantly, were taken up by the Nazi party in Germany before the Second World War.

eugenics
An outdated and totally wrong idea that the human gene pool could be cleaned up by removing faulty genes.

Old, erroneous ideas about the genetics of mental illness are illustrated by the following quotations. In Mein Kampf, Hitler said:

'Whoever is not bodily and spiritually healthy shall not have the right to pass on his suffering in the body of his children.'

Even Churchill, who is reputed to have suffered with depression himself, wrote in 1910:

'The unnatural and increasingly rapid growth of the feeble minded and insane classes, coupled as it is with steady restriction among all the thrifty, energetic and superior stocks, constitutes a national and race danger which it is impossible to exaggerate. I feel that the source from which the stream of madness is fed should be cut off and sealed before another year has passed.'

These ideas were deeply ingrained and stigmatizing.

Even if genes conferring susceptibility to schizophrenia were identified, it is extremely unlikely that anyone would recommend abortion for a foetus carrying a large number of these genes, because 'susceptibility' is by no means the same as 'definitely going to get it'. Far more likely, is that research in the future will be able to tell us how to prevent that susceptibility from leading to the illness, and so susceptible individuals will be given appropriate advice so as to avoid getting the illness. Other research is likely to lead to genetically tailored treatments.

Ideas about eugenics and the possibility of eliminating the genes for madness from the population led to a virtual holocaust of the mentally ill in Germany before the Second World War. The Nazis performed enforced sterilization and experimentation on the mentally ill. Their practices gave research into schizophrenia as a brain disorder, and genetic research in particular, a very bad name, which stuck for much of the latter part of the twentieth century. It was only after the 1980s, as new genetic techniques were developed, and we have been able to sequence and study our basic DNA, that the genetics of schizophrenia has become an important and untainted research topic once more.

The anti-genetic backlash (the nature-nurture debate) – yet more stigma for families

Ideas that schizophrenia could be caused by social factors alone, or was the result of poor parenting, or even that it was a myth and didn't exist at all, came about, in part, as a backlash to Nazi policies and the discredited eugenics movement of the early twentieth century. It is understandable, given what the Nazis did to the mentally ill, that there would be a post-war revulsion against anything 'genetic' or even 'scientific'. A sharp divide came about, on the one hand, between psychiatrists who continued to believe that schizophrenia was likely to be a biological, inherited brain disorder and, on the other, a group of more radical thinkers who felt schizophrenia was caused by social conditioning or family problems. This was known as the 'nature versus nurture' debate, 'nature' referring to genes, and 'nurture' referring to families and social environment.

my experience

Errol and Sam were unable to have children of their own. They were offered three children from the same family, in which both parents had schizophrenia. Errol and Sam were told that these children all had a 50:50 risk of developing the illness. They saw themselves as fortunate to be offered the chance to bring up these children and saw it as their task in life to give them the best home possible, and they educated themselves about schizophrenia in order to ensure their children had the latest treatment, if they did become ill. They said they found the knowledge they gained reassuring. When their oldest son became psychotic in his teens, Errol and Sam were well-prepared, and their son was treated early and has done well.

myth
Schizophrenia is caused by poor parenting

fact
Poor or even abusive parenting is not associated with
schizophrenia although these may lead to other problems in
adult life such as depression or personality disorder.

We now know that the cause of schizophrenia
is not 'nature' _or_ 'nurture' but 'nature' _and_
'nurture' interacting together.

The legacy of the 'anti-psychiatrists'

The post-war nature-nurture debate reached its
height in the 1960s and coincided with greater
social freedoms; it was the era of flower power,
free love and hallucinogenic drugs. The mood of
the day was to question authority and challenge
the establishment. Some challenges were helpful.
For example, the psychiatrist/philosopher R. D.
Laing criticized and rejected the poor conditions
patients had to endure in the mental hospitals of
the 1950s. Ken Kesey's book (and the later film)
One Flew Over the Cuckoo's Nest highlighted
these justified criticisms. The filming was set in a
real mental hospital, using real patients as well as
actors. Laing was also right when he told
psychiatrists to listen to their patients, rather than
ignoring what they said about their illness, which
was accepted teaching at the time. But in many
other ways Laing and the other anti-psychiatrists
were completely wrong, and their ideas were, in
their own way, as harmful and stigmatizing as
those of the Nazis.

Laing and the other anti-psychiatrists such as
Szasz saw schizophrenia as a social problem, if it

existed at all; they thought it was not genetic and not biological in any way. Laing saw poor parenting as the cause of schizophrenia; he had a very difficult relationship with his own parents and used them as an example in his writing. Others also believed that schizophrenia was a reaction to problems in the family. For example, Bateson had the idea of the **double bind** – he suggested that parents induced mental illness in their offspring by repeatedly placing them in intolerable situations.

double bind
An outdated and wrong idea that parents induce mental illness in their offspring by repeatedly placing them in intolerable situations.

myth
Schizophrenia can be triggered when parents put the child in 'double bind' situations.

fact
There is no evidence that any aspect of parenting leads to schizophrenia.

Some mothers were known as **schizophrenogenic** mothers because their parenting patterns were thought to have caused schizophrenia in their children.

schizophrenogenic
Causing schizophrenia, as in the term 'schizophrenogenic mother'. An old and discredited idea that the way a mother brings up a child can cause schizophrenia.

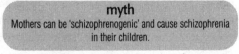

myth
Mothers can be 'schizophrenogenic' and cause schizophrenia in their children.

fact
This is an outdated idea. Upbringing does not cause schizophrenia.

Others went further and suggested that schizophrenia did not exist at all; psychiatric diagnoses were seen as 'labels'. Research into schizophrenia as a brain disorder was seen as 'propaganda'. The people who held these views were known as the 'anti-psychiatrists' and their influence continues today. For example, even today making a diagnosis of schizophrenia is sometimes dismissed as 'labelling', although the diagnosis of schizophrenia, clearly explained, carries with it the opportunity of appropriate support, information, treatment and recovery.

myth
Schizophrenia doesn't exist at all.

fact
Despite difficulties with diagnosis, the formal diagnosis of schizophrenia is helpful for psychiatrists in understanding and treating particular sets of symptoms, and this is true world-wide and for different cultures.

myth
Schizophrenia is a sane reaction to an insane world.

fact
The world can be a difficult and confusing place for all of us, but encouraging people who have a mental illness to think that they are well and just reacting rationally is likely to make them much worse and is likely to discourage them from getting the help they need.

The criticisms of the anti-psychiatrists grew to encompass all of psychiatry, which was considered repressive and insensitive to the rights of patients. Psychiatrists were seen as people seeking to control others, as seeking to crush the spirits of their patients, rather than help them. Psychiatry itself, as a profession, has suffered from its unpopular image. For decades, it has been an unpopular choice among medical students, although those with personal experience of mental illness in the family are more likely to choose it.

Even more harmful than the idea that schizophrenia did not exist, was the anti-psychiatrists' notion that the process of 'disintegration into psychosis' could actually be helpful and life-enhancing – psychosis was a 'choice' or a journey people needed to take. Hallucinogenic drugs were seen as offering positive and helpful experiences. Laing argued that people needed to be able to express their delusional ideas freely, because only in that way could they work through them, and achieve balance in their lives. But we now know that medical treatments *are* helpful and the earlier they are used, the better the final outcome will be. While the antipsychiatrists' views have almost entirely disappeared, there are still people around today who dismiss effective medical treatments for schizophrenia as rubbish.

myth
Psychiatric diagnosis is merely labelling.

fact
The diagnosis of schizophrenia has been refined over decades of psychiatric practice and describes a known pattern of behaviour that occurs when certain parts of the brain are involved. It is wrong and unhelpful to suggest that the diagnosis has just been 'made up' as a convenient way of controlling difficult people, as argued by some anti-psychiatrists.

my experience

John was born a twin in 1950, but his twin brother, David, died at the age of ten. John developed schizophrenia in the late 1960s and had visual hallucinations centred on a wart on his hand. He had visual and auditory hallucinations of his dead brother watching and talking to him from the wart. The therapist considered that John's hallucinations were an appropriate and helpful response to the disordered family dynamics which had arisen after David's death, and John was encouraged to 'work through' his psychosis. He was not admitted to hospital or offered medication. John found the hallucinations unbearable and cut his hand off by placing it on a railway line.

Luckily, ideas that having schizophrenia is helpful, and should be 'worked through' without treatment, are seldom encountered nowadays. But there are still people who hold the simplistic notion that family dynamics is the basis for psychosis, and who reject outright any biological influence.

my experience

Bob and Angie were unable to have children of their own. In the 1980s they adopted Jason. Both Jason's biological parents had schizophrenia, but Bob and Angie were told by the social worker (who held views that were old-fashioned even for that time) that schizophrenia was not genetic at all. The social worker said that schizophrenia was the result of disordered communication in the family, so there was no way the child would become schizophrenic like his biological parents if he was brought up by 'good' parents like themselves. Sadly, Jason did develop schizophrenia. (We now know that his risk was 45–50 per cent, because both biological parents had the illness.) Bob and Angie's initial reaction was guilt, then, as they learned the true facts about the genetic inheritance of schizophrenia, they reacted with anger and disappointment. Their feelings led them to reject Jason. The team caring for Jason felt that his illness was made much worse because of the rejection by his adoptive parents.

The notion that schizophrenia is simply a reaction to problems in the family is deeply stigmatizing and very harmful. It is bad enough to try to cope with a son or daughter who has become mentally ill, but how much worse if you are told that it is your fault, that you have induced mental illness in your offspring by placing them 'double binds' as Bateson hypothesized, repeatedly placing them in intolerable situations. Countless mothers are still tormented, to this day, by these stigmatizing ideas – or perhaps by the suggestion, often unspoken, that they are responsible for their child's schizophrenia.

Of course, families where one member has schizophrenia may indeed be dysfunctional, but the anti-psychiatrists did not appear to consider that the family may have become that way because of the difficulty of dealing with the psychotic family member.

Current thinking about schizophrenia and the family

Some useful statistics

As discussed previously (Chapter 3) there is a considerable genetic predisposition to developing schizophrenia. Overall, looking at an entire population, the percentage 'cause' of schizophrenia that could be considered 'genetic' is around 80 per cent. The genes involved may act in different ways, for example, they may influence the chemical or anatomical structure of the brain, others may confer susceptibility to the effect of drugs such as cannabis or another hallucinogen.

The 80 per cent heritability of schizophrenia is derived from looking at the rates of schizophrenia in various groups of relatives. If one parent has the disorder, then the child has a 13 per cent risk but if both parents are schizophrenic, then the child has a 45–50 per cent risk. The risk to a sibling of a brother or sister with schizophrenia is 10–13 per cent and the risk to more distant relatives, such as grandparents, grandchildren, aunts, uncles, nephews and nieces is around three per cent. The importance of 'non-genetic' factors is illustrated by the risk figures for twins. If one member of an identical twin pair has schizophrenia, then the other twin has a 50 per cent risk of developing the illness, whereas if it were fully genetic, the risk would be 100 per cent for the identical twin because they are genetically identical.

These numbers may seem high, if you feel you are on 'the receiving end' of these risk statistics. But consider how common schizophrenia is in the general population – one per cent of *everyone* will be affected. Then consider other common illnesses such as depression, which affects 15 per cent of the population, dementia which affects six per cent of people over the age of 65 or cancer where 25 per cent of us will die of the disease, not to mention common problems such as heart disease, diabetes, accidental injury or infections. People sometimes say they feel more comfortable with the risk of other common illnesses, but this is usually because they know more about them.

Genetic counselling for mental disorders is available in some specialized centres. This can address many different concerns such as: 'My son has schizophrenia. How likely are his children to have it?' 'I am thinking of adopting a child whose mother had schizophrenia. How likely is the child also to suffer from the disorders?'

genetic counselling
Counselling about the risk to a family member of occurrence of a genetic disorder (or partly genetic disorder, such as schizophrenia).

High expressed emotion and schizophrenia

It is well known that the response of the family can influence the course of an illness in a family member, but people seldom stop to think of the difficulties encountered by that family, or how the presence of someone who is unwell can influence the behaviour of everyone else. Nevertheless, however they come about, negative attitudes in the family are associated with a poorer outcome.

The statement that family attitudes can influence the course of an illness is not the same as saying that they *caused* the illness. The general term 'illness' is used here deliberately. The finding that family responses may influence the course of the illness is true whether the illness is diabetes, anorexia nervosa, chronic fatigue syndrome, acne or schizophrenia.

The psychiatrist Julian Leff found that three separate 'attitudes' among families have a negative effect on outcome in schizophrenia. They are:

◇ criticism (statements of dislike, resentment or annoyance)
◇ hostility (statements indicating rejection and general criticism of the ill individual as a person)
◇ emotional overinvolvement (over-protectiveness, over-concern and self-sacrificing attitudes).

Families can be categorized into 'high' and 'low' EE (expressed emotion). It is thought that high EE is associated with poor self-esteem, depression and rejection of the diagnosis by family members, and it is important to identify families where this is a problem, because people with schizophrenia from families where there is high expressed emotion tend to relapse more frequently (the relapse rates may be almost double in high EE environments). It is thought that these relapses may be due to higher levels of anxiety and depression in the sufferer.

Fortunately, families can learn to overcome high EE tendencies. **Family therapy**, where a therapist sees all the family members together and helps them to understand any negative attitudes, can be very useful.

family therapy
A therapy designed to alter negative attitudes, expectations and communication within a family where there is a psychiatrically ill member.

Carers can also learn how to reduce any highly charged emotional responses to the person with schizophrenia and to modify their behaviour to be as helpful as possible. There are courses run by the charity, Rethink, and the carers can then pass on their learning to new carers, in turn.

myth
High expressed emotion in families is specific to schizophrenia.

fact
High expressed emotion is common in families who are caring for an ill family member and this is true for most illnesses, including diabetes and even acne.

If a member of your family has schizophrenia you should avoid:

✧ family arguments about the problems caused by the illness
✧ hostile and critical comments
✧ fussing too much
✧ obvious self-sacrifice.

Effects on children of parents with schizophrenia

Does being brought up by someone with schizophrenia cause problems in the child? Research has shown us that having a biological parent with schizophrenia raises the risk for schizophrenia in the child, but the risk seems to be genetic, rather than anything to do with upbringing. Nevertheless, many parents with schizophrenia experience the sadness and stress of having their child removed and fostered or adopted away because they are unable to cope with parenting.

Once the baby is born, someone with schizophrenia *can* have difficulties rearing the child, even if there is no active psychotic illness at the time. If the schizophrenic illness is severe, the parent may be unable to show sufficient attention or emotional warmth towards the baby and this can lead to the baby's failure to thrive. Because early influences are extremely important to the child's development, it is important that the mother-child relationship, and the child's physical, social and emotional needs are monitored.

my experience

Darren and Kathy met on a hospital ward. They developed a relationship which lasted through several further admissions for each of them; both were diagnosed with schizophrenia. Darren and Kathy functioned well as a couple. Both were treated with depot injections of antipsychotic medication. (This has a contraceptive effect because of alterations in hormone levels.) Kathy was then changed to a different medication, clozapine, which does not have any effect on hormone levels, and within six months she fell pregnant.

Darren and Kathy were keen to keep their baby, and Kathy was admitted to a mother and baby unit, where her parenting skills were considered good enough to allow her to go home with the baby. The family was closely monitored. Sadly, within a few weeks of going home, the baby stopped growing and putting on weight, and the social worker noticed that the baby wasn't gurgling or making eye contact and her activity levels had reduced. The baby was clean and was being fed, but neither Darren nor Kathy were able to pay sufficient attention to the baby's emotional needs, and this was causing a failure to thrive. The decision was eventually taken by all concerned that the baby should be cared for by Kathy's mother.

clozapine
An antipsychotic for treatment-resistant schizophrenia. Requires ongoing blood testing for risk of neutropenia.

It must be remembered that Darren and Kathy were both very unwell. In many other cases one or both parents have milder cases of the illness and manage to bring up their families without difficulty. There is no evidence that being brought up by someone who has schizophrenia leads to any greater risk for the child having the illness themselves.

> **my experience**
>
> Karen came to the clinic with worries about her teenage son. She explained that her mother had schizophrenia and had been admitted to hospital on several occasions during Karen's childhood. The mother's illness eventually led to divorce. Karen and her brother Trevor were cared for by their grandmother for quite long periods while their mother was in hospital. However, both Karen and Trevor grew up to be successful adults with a positive view of family life, a deep bond with their mother and considerable respect for her ability to carry on despite her illness.

Conclusions

✧ Views about psychiatry in the 1960s, typified by the 'anti-psychiatrists', led to mistaken views about the role of the family in schizophrenia.

✧ Upbringing does not cause schizophrenia.

✧ When a person does have schizophrenia, it is important that emotional stress in family life is avoided.

✧ The only situation where the genetic risk of having a child with schizophrenia would be considered high enough to warrant caution about having a family, is where both parents have the illness.

✧ Children brought up by a parent with schizophrenia are at no increased risk of developing schizophrenia themselves, by reason of their upbringing alone.

CHAPTER

5 Treatments for schizophrenia

There are a variety of treatments used for schizophrenia, which are laid out in the NICE (National Institute of Clinical Excellence) guidelines for the disorder, published in 2002. These guidelines were developed with the advice of service users, carers, mental health charities, as well as various mental health professionals, and the evidence upon which they were based was also provided. Clinical guidelines are extremely helpful to both clinicians and the people receiving the treatments.

Medication

There are three main groups of medication used in schizophrenia: antipsychotic medication, antidepressant medication and mood stabilizers.

Antipsychotic medication

Antipsychotic medication is, as the name implies, used for the treatment of psychosis. It is remarkably effective, and works by influencing or blocking the action of certain chemicals in the brain. Brain cells communicate with each other using these chemicals (known as neurotransmitters). Different chemicals are active in different parts of the brain. We have seen in previous chapters that the neurotransmitter dopamine, which is found in the **limbic system** (which governs sensation and emotion), is involved in psychotic symptoms. Chapter 3 outlines the relevant research in more detail.

> ### limbic system
> The area of the brain involved in sensation and emotion. When the connections in the limbic area of the brain are faulty, errors develop in the ability to process information about the outside world and about ourselves, and this is known as 'psychosis'.

For the past 50 years antipsychotic medication has been available which reduces the action of dopamine in the brain. The medication does this by sticking on to the ends of the cells which use dopamine as a neurotransmitter, so blocking their action. This improves psychotic symptoms. There are several different kinds of dopamine receptors which may be blocked by different medication and these receptors are blocked to different degrees. Other neurotransmitters are also involved, and there is medication which also blocks these.

Dopamine is also used as a neurotransmitter in other parts of the brain. This is why it causes unwanted side effects. For example, dopamine is used in the body movement part of the brain, particularly the part that goes wrong when someone develops Parkinsonism. For this reason, some of the unwanted effects of antipsychotic medication are called **Parkinsonian side effects** and involve abnormal movements, stiffness or tremor.

> ### Parkinsonian side effects
> Side effects of antipsychotic medication that involve abnormal movements, stiffness or tremor.

> ### serotonin
> A neurotransmitter thought to be involved in psychosis. Some medication inhibits the reuptake of serotonin.

Another neurotransmitter, **serotonin** (known as $5-HT_2$), is also thought to be involved in psychosis. We know that stimulation of serotonin-releasing brain cells by substances like amphetamine or LSD causes hallucinations. Serotonin is also involved in mood, and depression is associated with low levels of serotonin. Serotonin is important for the sleep/wake cycle and the serotonin system and the dopamine system are interactive.

Antipsychotic medication – the choices

Antipsychotics treat psychotic symptoms, and they are very effective in up to 80 per cent of people with schizophrenia. However, choosing the right medication is not straightforward because different people respond to different medication in different ways, particularly with regard to side effects. The decision about medication should be taken *jointly* by the prescriber and the person taking the medication, who should be informed about the potential side effects and the choices they have. There may be some situations when someone is so acutely ill that discussion is not possible, but it should always take place once the person is well enough.

Antipsychotics can be divided into two types, the older typical antipsychotics (called 'typical' because they 'typically' block dopamine cell receptors and 'typically' cause certain side effects), and the newer atypical antipsychotics, so called because their mode of action is more complex, and side effects may be less of a problem.

The NICE guidelines have made certain broad recommendations. NICE guidance has recommended that atypical antipsychotics should be the first choice among people who have

Q What are the forms in which psychiatric medication can be given?

A Tablets, a liquid, long-acting depot injections lasting two to six weeks or short acting injections lasting hours or days.

newly diagnosed schizophrenia, or in any person who is acutely ill where discussion with the person is not possible. Atypical antipsychotics should also be given when someone is suffering unacceptable side effects from a typical antipsychotic.

Typical antipsychotics should be continued in individuals who are already on a typical antipsychotic and who do not suffer unacceptable side effects. They are also used in emergency situations, and in individuals who require depot (long-acting) antipsychotics.

Side effects are not the only area where medication choice is required. Antipsychotic medication also differs in the degree of *sedation* it causes. If someone is having trouble sleeping, then a sedative antipsychotic can be a real benefit. There is also choice about the form in which the medication can be taken. Antipsychotics can be given in a number of forms: tablets, liquid, long-acting **depot** injections lasting two to six weeks, or short-acting injections lasting hours or days.

Nearly all medication causes unwanted effects. Some unwanted effects are very rare, others more common. If you think you are experiencing a side effect, it is best to discuss it with your doctor. *Don't just stop the medication*. This can sometimes lead to withdrawal effects or a return of the illness.

The newer 'atypical' medications are much more expensive than the older drugs. The prescriber's choice of medication should *never* be made on the basis of cost, although examples of more appropriate (but more expensive) medication being withheld on the ground of cost were widespread before the NICE guidelines

depot medication
Slow release medication given by injection.

Q Who should be given the new atypical antipsychotics?

A People with newly diagnosed schizophrenia, people who are acutely unwell and who cannot discuss the options, and people suffering unacceptable side effects.

came into force, and some of these problems may persist.

Antipsychotic medication – unwanted effects

The choice of medication often involves a discussion about which side effects the person is likely to tolerate most easily. People differ in their tendency to suffer side effects.

All antipsychotics *can* cause a very wide range of side effects. It is important to remember that any medication can cause unusual or idiosyncratic side effects in some people, so it is important to consult the prescriber if there is any worry at all. The following side effects are those that are typically seen, but there is a more detailed list of side effects in the British National Formulary.

Overall, antipsychotic medication is remarkably safe. Although the standard advice about any medication (for any medical condition) is to stop taking it if you are pregnant, antipsychotic medication is generally safe in pregnancy, although your doctor should always be consulted.

Extra pyramidal side effects (EPSEs – sometimes known as Parkinsonian side effects

EPSEs occur because the dopamine-using brain cells in a certain part of the brain are blocked, including the part of the brain (the nigro-striatal system) which is also affected in Parkinson's disease (hence the name 'Parkinsonian side effects'). These side effects are nearly always reversible, but can, occasionally, be permanent. They are particularly frequent with the older

Q What should I do if I think medication is being 'rationed' on the grounds of cost?

A Complain. Contact a support organization such as Rethink.

EPSEs (extrapyramidal side effects)
Side effects of particularly the older typical antipsychotic medication which can include movement problems such as tremors, restlessness, muscle spasms, and a shuffling gait, as well as a wide range of other problems. Also seen to a lesser extent with some newer atypical drugs.

typical antipsychotic drugs. Studies suggest that up to 80 per cent of individuals on typical antipsychotics will have EPSEs.

Reversible EPSEs

Reversible EPSEs include:

✧ Dystonic reaction (acute cramp-like muscle spasms and stiffness affecting any voluntary muscle group including the eye muscles). This usually happens when the medication is given for the first time.
✧ Dystonia (sustained cramp-like abnormalities of posture associated with muscle stiffness).
✧ Akathisia (a sense of restlessness in the muscles and inability to sit still).
✧ Parkinsonian symptoms: rhythmic tremor (typically affecting mouth, tongue, arms and hands), immobility of the muscles (leading to loss of facial expression and slow body movements).

EPSEs can be treated with a drug such as procyclidine or orphenadrine, or a beta blocker (propranolol). However nowadays, it is probably better to switch to a different antipsychotic.

Possible irreversible EPSEs

These are among the most worrying side effects of the antipsychotic drugs, although they are rare. Tardive dyskinesia is a permanent tremor, or dystonic movement disorder. This may occur if side effects which are ordinarily reversible are simply treated with long-term anti-Parkinsonian medication while the drug itself, which caused the problem, is left unchanged. Switching to certain atypical antipsychotic drugs, such as clozapine or quetiapine, may be beneficial.

A cautionary tale: Sharon had well-controlled schizophrenia. She had been taking a depot antipsychotic once a month for several years, and she was doing very well. Sharon was able to work, drive a car and had a stable relationship. Sharon complained of attacks of 'blindness' which seemed to occur on a monthly basis, often when she was driving her car; she had to pull over onto the hard shoulder and wait for it to pass, which it always did. She went to her ophthalmologist and nothing was found to be wrong with her eyes. After some detective work, her GP wondered if the attacks had anything to do with her depot medication. Sharon's husband then confirmed that he had seen Sharon's eyes 'go up into her head' if she was stressed or anxious, particularly in the days just after the depot had been given. Sharon said she was often anxious and stressed when driving. The psychiatrist confirmed that Sharon was having acute dystonic reactions affecting her eyes. All EPSEs can be worse in stressful circumstances. Her medication was changed to an atypical drug which did not cause EPSEs, and the problem was solved!

Anticholinergic (muscarinic) side effects

These occur because the medications attach to certain cell receptors in the body call 'muscarinic' receptors. They include:

- ✧ rapid heart rate
- ✧ dry mouth
- ✧ inability or difficulty urinating
- ✧ constipation
- ✧ blurred vision.

These side effects usually wear off and are not generally severe enough to warrant stopping the medication.

Anti-adrenergic side effects

These include a drop in blood pressure when standing up suddenly (postural hypotension) and inhibition of ejaculation. These side effects usually wear off, and are not usually severe enough to warrant stopping the medication.

Side effects associated with increased prolactin hormone

Prolactin is a naturally occurring hormone (found in both men and women) which rises in pregnancy and causes breast enlargement and milk production. A rise in prolactin is also associated with reductions in libido and fertility.

> **prolactin**
> A naturally occurring hormone in men and women involved in normal sexual functioning and pregnancy.

Most typical antipsychotic drugs, and some of the newer atypicals, cause a rise in prolactin levels to ten times normal levels or more. This is a 'silent' side effect; the first many women know about it is that their menstrual periods stop or become irregular (up to 90 per cent will have this side effect). Other side effects are decreased libido in men and women, impotence and or erectile failure in men (25–50 per cent). Both men and women can suffer breast tenderness, enlargement and milk production. There may also be a tendency to acne or even excessive hairiness. In some people there may even be a tendency to anxiety and depression. One of the most worrying problems is the association of high levels of prolactin with reduced bone density (osteoporosis) in the long term for both men and women.

These side effects are often ignored or minimized by prescribers, but can cause significant distress in people taking the medication.

Effects on the heart

Fast heart beat, changes in the electrical conduction of the heart (tested with an electrocardiogram or ECG), or myocarditis – an inflammation of the heart muscle.

Weight gain

Weight gain occurs because the medication causes the person to feel hungry and to eat more. It can be a problem with all antipsychotic drugs, but it is difficult to predict which individuals are likely to be affected, and by how much. Some very strong minded people avoid weight gain entirely, by limiting their intake and joining a gym, and other people just don't seem to put on weight, but these are the exceptions. For most people weight gain is a serious issue.

Clozapine is associated with the greatest amount of weight gain. However, the advantages of this medication more than make up for the side effects. If clozapine leads to a recovery from the illness, then that person is likely to become sufficiently motivated to be able to engage in a weight loss programme, increase their exercise levels and improve their diet.

Olanzapine and zotepine are also associated with weight gain and, to a greater or less extent, so are all typical antipsychotics. Aripiprazole, an atypical antipsychotic, does not appear to cause weight gain in most people and this may be a reason for its popularity. There is another atypical medication (ziprasidone) which does not cause weight gain, but this is not available in the UK.

Metabolic problems

For reasons which are as yet undiscovered, people with schizophrenia who have never taken any medication, are more likely to have diabetes. Antipsychotics may further increase the risk of diabetes, particularly those that cause weight gain. Clozapine and olanzapine are particularly likely to be associated with diabetes.

Other side effects

Almost anything is possible! Remember to consult your doctor if you have any worries. Side effects can usually be managed by a switch to an alternative antipsychotic. Less common side effects include allergic or photosensitive skin reactions, pigment changes in the skin, liver problems, reduction in white cell count in the blood, epileptic seizures, nausea and agitation.

Depot or tablets?

Long-acting depot injections have been available since the 1960s. They are promoted as a useful way of helping people to stay on their medication, when they might otherwise stop taking it. Psychiatrists in the UK are particularly likely to prescribe depots, compared to their European counterparts. Studies have shown that many patients prefer the convenience of depots. The medication is given as an injection once every two to six weeks (usually once a month).

There are advantages and disadvantages to depot medication. The NICE guidelines suggest that medication decisions should be taken jointly by the prescriber and the patient, and it is important to consider the decision to use a depot in detail. Most depots are typical antipsychotics, and share their disadvantages in terms of EPSE and prolactin related side effects, although there is at least one atypical depot (risperidone).

Unwanted effects may be a particular problem with a medication that stays in the body for long periods of time. Other disadvantages relate to the depot itself; this requires a deep intramuscular injection into the buttock, which some people find unpleasant. On the other hand, some people enjoy the freedom from tablet taking offered by depot injections.

'Typical' antipsychotic medication

Side effects may be more troublesome with the typical antipsychotic drugs, particularly EPSEs. These drugs can be subdivided into three broad groups on the basis of their sedative effects and side effects.

(NB *Drugs have a compound name and a trade (manufacturer's) name which always starts with a capital letter.*)

✧ **Group 1 phenothiazines** – include: chlorpromazine (Largactil), levomepromazine (Nozinan), promazine (Promazine) and are more *sedative*. They carry a moderate likelihood of antimuscarinic side effects and EPSEs.

⋄ **Group 2 phenothiazines** – include: pericyazine (Neulactil) and pipothiazine (Piportil) which are only moderately sedative, but have marked antimuscarinic effects, and are less likely to cause EPSEs than groups 1 or 3.

⋄ **Group 3 phenothiazines and other typical drugs** – include: fluphenazine (Modecate), perphenazine (Fentazin), prochlorperazine (Stemetil), trifluoperazine (Stelazine) benperidol (Benquil), haloperidol, (Haldol, Serenace, Haldol Decanoate), pimozide* (Orap), flupentixol (Fluanxol, Depixol), zuclopenthixol (Clopixol) and sulpiride (Dolmatil, Sulpitil, Sulpor). These drugs are more likely to cause EPSEs but have fewer sedative effects and fewer antimuscarinic effects than groups 1 and 2.

(*People taking this medication should have an annual ECG test of the heart, and care should be taken when combining with other medication.)

'Atypical' antipsychotic medication

Atypical antipsychotics are so-called because they do *not* typically produce EPSEs as often as atypical drugs. However, although EPSEs are much less likely with atypicals, they *can* occur with any of them. Some atypicals (aripiprazole, clozapine and quetiapine) cause minimal or no rise in prolactin. Overall, there is much greater variability in the chemical characteristics of the atypicals, compared to typical antipsychotics, and this can lead to some idiosyncratic side effects. Atypicals are at least as effective as typical antipsychotics, and some studies suggest that the relapse rate is lower with people taking atypicals.

There are other possible benefits from the atypical antipsychotics. Some have an effect on negative symptoms, some improve cognitive impairment, and others help with mood, either improving depression or stabilizing the mood.

Clozapine is the only medication, typical or atypical, that has been shown to be of very significant benefit for negative symptoms. This claim has been made for some other atypicals, such as aripiprazole, risperidone, olanzapine and quetiapine, but the effect is less striking. Clozapine also improves cognitive impairment. Quetiapine and risperidone may also have some effect on cognitive symptoms. Olanzapine also acts as a mood stabilizer (and has been licensed for this use) as well as having an antidepressant effect.

Atypical antipsychotics are often better tolerated in terms of side effects. However, weight gain is a particular problem with some atypical antipsychotics, which may be otherwise low in side effects. Remember, any medication can cause unusual or idiosyncratic side effects in some people, so it is important to consult the prescriber if there is any worry at all. A full list of side effects is found in the British National Formulary.

Atypical antipsychotic medication includes the following drugs:

- ✧ **amisulpride (Solian)** – causes raised prolactin levels and can sometimes cause EPSEs. It can also cause insomnia. Weight gain is less of a problem.
- ✧ **aripiprazole (Abilify)** – can most often cause nausea, anxiety, vomiting and

insomnia, and sometimes EPSE, particularly akathisia. It is not associated with weight gain or with prolactin elevation.

◇ **olanzapine (Zyprexa)** – can most often cause sedation, weight gain, some anti-muscarinic effects such as constipation, some risk of EPSEs and a transient rise in prolactin (not usually a serious problem).

◇ **quetiapine (Seroquel)** – can most often cause postural hypotension (low blood pressure when getting up suddenly), sedation, dry mouth, weight gain, constipation, and heart conduction problems. There is little or no risk of EPSEs with quetiapine, and for this reason it is useful for people who already have a movement disorder, or who are at high risk. There is also little or no risk of prolactin elevation.

◇ **risperidone (Risperdal)** – can most often cause low blood pressure when getting up suddenly, raised prolactin levels, EPSEs, insomnia, agitation, headaches and sexual dysfunction. Risperidone can be given as a depot preparation, but this is more difficult to administer than typical antipsychotic depots.

◇ **sertindole (Serdolect)** – was taken off the market for a time because of its effect on heart conduction. Its use is restricted to patients enroled in clinical studies who are intolerant of at least one other antipsychotic. It can cause dry mouth, low blood pressure when getting up suddenly and nasal congestion. It is not likely to cause sedation or EPSEs and has little effect on prolactin.

◇ **zotepine (Zoleptil)** – can most often cause sedation, prolactin elevation, low blood pressure when getting up suddenly, heart conduction problems and weight gain. There is some risk of EPSEs.

✧ **clozapine (Clozaril, Denzapine, Zaponex)** – deserves special consideration, because it is a medication like no other. It is reserved for people with schizophrenia whose illness is unresponsive to other medications or if they cannot tolerate other medication. It can only be taken in tablet form.

Clozapine – a special case

NICE suggests that clozapine should be introduced at the earliest opportunity in patients whose illness has not responded to sequential use of two different antipsychotics at therapeutic dose (one of which must be atypical) for six to eight weeks each.

Clozapine can lead to remarkable improvement in symptoms and, sometimes, a complete recovery for people who might otherwise be chronically unwell. Clozapine is unusual in many ways. First, it is unclear exactly how it works and why it is so effective; second, it has an unusual range of side effects, third, clozapine takes up to a year to work, and fourth, clozapine is perhaps the only antipsychotic that has a marked effect on the negative symptoms of schizophrenia.

Clozapine is not likely to cause prolactin elevation or EPSEs. It can cause one or more of the following: weight gain, excess salivation, low blood pressure when getting up suddenly and constipation.

Clozapine was initially brought out in the 1970s and was soon realized to be extremely effective not only on positive (psychotic) symptoms, but

neutropenia

A condition in which there is a reduced number of neutrophils in white blood count. This can be a consequence of drug treatment, particularly, but not exclusively, clozapine. It is a requirement of taking clozapine that ongoing testing for this is undertaken.

also on negative symptoms. However, there were a number of deaths because of a lowering of the white cells of the blood (known as **neutropenia**), and clozapine was taken off the market. Drug companies then attempted to find a drug as good as clozapine without this side effect, but they failed. It was felt that the significant benefits of clozapine outweighed the risk of this side effect as long as regular checks were made on the white count, and clozapine was brought back in 1989. The risk of neutropenia declines the longer clozapine is taken, and the risk is around 1 per cent of patients in the first year of use.

Clozapine is a difficult drug to take. It must be started at a low dose and then gradually brought up to avoid other side effects such as low blood pressure and fast heart beat. It is very prone to cause constipation, and nearly always causes weight gain and sometimes diabetes. Clozapine often causes an increase in salivation and sometimes a tendency to wet the bed at night. Another possible side effect is a disorder of the heart (cardiomyopathy, or myocarditis).

However, the most important side effect of clozapine is neutropenia (lowering of the white cell count in the blood). For this reason, white cell counts must be normal before starting clozapine and must be checked regularly thereafter. They are checked weekly for 18 weeks then every two weeks and, after one year, white counts are checked monthly.

You might think, reading this, that taking clozapine is not likely to be worth while, and perhaps not the drug for you or someone close to you, but it is well worth the effort – clozapine is uniquely effective.

Clozapine is reserved for people with schizophrenia whose illness has not responded to two other antipsychotic drugs. For people in this situation (sometimes known as 'treatment resistant'), clozapine can be a life changing medication. Once the initial stages are over, the side effects of clozapine generally settle, or can be managed with other medication. The success rate for recovery from schizophrenia is high, and better the earlier clozapine is given. Overall, the way the drug is regarded by prescribers and, more importantly, by the people taking clozapine is overwhelmingly positive.

There is a final note of caution. At the time of writing, there is no other medication either on the market, or in the pipeline, which has clozapine's unique effect on schizophrenia. People who stop clozapine to try a new drug usually experience a return of their symptoms and become very unwell.

my experience

A clozapine success story: Libby was unusually young (only 13) when she developed schizophrenia. There was a strong family history of schizophrenia, as her father, and his brother, both had the illness. Libby started to use cannabis at school, and within a few months she had begun to feel paranoid and anxious. Libby responded to this by using more cannabis, and stopping school. By the age of 14 she was acutely psychotic and completely out of touch with reality. She thought angels and devils were guiding her; she could feel, hear, touch and see them. Libby would wander out of the house at night, trying to follow the angels, or get away from the devils. Her mother was distraught and took to locking the house but, when she did this, Libby would shout and kick at the door and, on one occasion, broke a window to get out of the house and cut herself badly.

Libby was admitted to an inpatient adolescent unit, where she was tried on an atypical antipsychotic medication. Over the next few months, she became calmer, and gained about two-and-a-half stones in weight, but her delusions and hallucinations concerning the angels and devils continued, and she was very unwilling to take the medication and would try to hide the tablets in her clothes. Libby was then tried on a depot injection, but this did not help her symptoms, and there was a frightening incident when she absconded from hospital and was found on the motorway at night by a 'good samaritan' who took her to the police station in his own car. Libby's mother was terrified when she thought about the kind of person who might have found Libby. Finally, six months after her admission, and after a second opinion from a visiting psychiatrist, Libby was started on clozapine.

The first six months on clozapine were very hard for Libby. She had such bad excess salivation that her pillows were soaked with saliva in the morning. She gained another stone in weight and appeared sedated. However, gradually, things started to change. Libby lost her psychotic symptoms and was able to go home on the weekends. Within two months of starting clozapine Libby was discharged home. She stayed on the medication because she felt so relieved to have lost her hallucinations. Libby and her mother joined a gym. By the time she was 16, Libby was able to go to college to catch up on her school work. She eventually took an NVQ in care of the elderly and got a job in an old people's home.

At the age of 20 Libby had a job, a boyfriend, and a new baby. By this time she had been on clozapine for nearly five years, including throughout her pregnancy. Her weight continued to be a problem, particularly after having the baby, but Libby has remained psychiatrically well, working, and caring for her family. She has no plans to stop the medication and she and her mother have had to argue her case to stay on it with the adult mental health team, who agreed only after they obtained all the records from the adolescent unit.

Stopping antipsychotic medication

A useful rule of thumb adopted by most prescribers is to ask the person who has psychosis to continue their medication for one full year after the psychotic symptoms have stopped. If the medication is carefully withdrawn after this time, and the symptoms recur, then it should be taken for between two and five years. If there is a further relapse after another attempt to stop, then the person should be encouraged to take the medication indefinitely. Taking medication for long periods involves careful monitoring of side effects and the physical health of the person taking it.

Clozapine is, again, in a different category. First, it takes up to a year to work in any case, second, improvements with clozapine can increase, year on year, and third, the side effects tend to decrease the longer it is taken. Clozapine is unusual in that there can be a relapse after stopping clozapine within a matter of days, unlike other medication. Most importantly, if there is a relapse when clozapine is stopped, it can take *several years* for the same level of improvement to return, and *a similar degree of recovery may never return*.

Other forms of medication

Antidepressants

Antidepressants are always given as tablets or liquid. There are many more antidepressants on the market than antipsychotics. Most people with schizophrenia will be offered an antidepressant at some stage of their illness, because depression frequently accompanies schizophrenia.

Antidepressants are divided into main groups; older **tricyclic** antidepressants (so-called because of their chemical structure) such as amitriptyline, clomipramine, dothiepin, doxepin, imipramine and lofepramine may have similar

tricyclics
One of the major classes of antidepressants, so classified because of their structure.

anticholinergic side effects to some of the antipsychotic drugs, so such problems as constipation may occur. Nowadays the most frequently prescribed antidepressants are **SSRIs** (serotonin specific reuptake inhibitors), which include citalopram, escitalopram, fluoxetine, fluvoxamine, paroxetine and sertraline. These medications tend to be safer and better tolerated than the tricyclics, but they can cause side effects including nausea, dizziness and sexual dysfunction.

> ### SSRIs (serotonin – specific reuptake inhibitors)
> One of the major classes of antidepressant medications. Includes prozac (fluoxetine).

Some of these drugs have become controversial because they can cause agitation, which can in turn lead to suicidal thoughts. They can also cause very unpleasant side effects if they are stopped too rapidly. There are many other antidepressants which are used in certain situations, particularly venlafaxine, which is effective in resistant depression. It is always best, if you are prescribed a medication, to ask why it is being given, why the prescriber is recommending one particular drug over another, and what are the most common side effects.

Mood stabilizers

People with schizophrenia may be offered mood stabilizers to augment the antipsychotic medication, or if mood is a particular problem. There are five in common use: lithium, carbamazepine, valproate, lamotrigine and gabapentin. Lithium is unique in its action and can have quite marked side effects such as thirst, frequent urination (and a kind of diabetes associated with this), tremor, acne, muscular weakness, weight gain and effects on the thyroid and kidneys. The usual dose of lithium is quite close to the toxic dose, so it must be carefully checked with a blood level of lithium, usually every three to six months.

The other mood stabilizers mentioned are all used, primarily, as anti-epileptic drugs. Drowsiness is a problem with carbamazepine and valproate, but is not so much of a problem with lamotrigine. All can cause headache and nausea and some are contra-indicated in combination with particular antipsychotics (e.g. carbamazepine should never be given with clozapine).

Diet and essential fatty acids

There were high hopes a few years ago that omega-3 fatty acids (found in oily fish and linseeds, for example) would be of benefit in schizophrenia. The research has not been altogether positive, as the studies done so far suggest that omega-3 fatty acids do not lead to any dramatic reduction in the symptoms of schizophrenia, although they are of benefit in depression. However, an adequate intake of omega-3 fatty acids is good for many general health reasons, because it protects against coronary heart disease and various inflammatory conditions.

Therapies

Cognitive behavioural therapy

Cognitive behavioural therapy (CBT) has been used for depression for several decades. It is used to break the cycle of negative thoughts associated with depression. More recently, CBT has been developed for psychosis and schizophrenia, and focuses directly on core

cognitive behavioural therapy
Use of cognitive and behavioural techniques to change behaviours, attitudes and negative ways of thinking (e.g. 'I'll always fail', 'I'll always be rejected') with strategies designed to encourage suitable behaviour and positive ways of thinking, thereby boosting self-esteem. A form of cognitive therapy can be helpful in schizophrenia to help individuals cope with and control psychotic symptoms.

psychotic symptoms such as delusions or hallucinations. In CBT for psychosis, people with schizophrenia are trained to take responsibility for, and control of their psychotic experiences with the help of their therapist.

It is important to have a trusting relationship with the therapist for CBT for psychosis to work and establishing this relationship is the first step in therapy. The goal of therapy is to reduce the distress which accompanies delusional beliefs or hallucinations. The truth/existence (or not) of the belief or hallucination is not an initial focus of therapy. The therapist aims to establish strategies to deal with these stressful symptoms, such as relaxation, sleep, engaging in an activity and other forms of distraction. A further strand in the therapy is to encourage the individual to weigh evidence to contradict delusional beliefs and also to evaluate negative beliefs about themselves. The pace of the sessions takes into account problems that individuals may have with cognitive impairment; the therapist asks for feedback, and provides written information (based on previous sessions) for the patient to read between sessions.

Not everyone with schizophrenia can manage CBT for psychosis. There has to be a willingness to embark on therapy and sufficient cognitive ability to understand and work with the techniques offered.

Family therapy

Families are the most consistent factor in people's lives. Most people who are discharged after a psychiatric admission to hospital return to their families, or remain in close contact with them. In Chapter 4 we saw that high expressed emotion (criticism, hostility and emotional over-involvement) can contribute to relapse. Fortunately, family members can learn techniques to reduce high expressed emotion. They are provided with education about schizophrenia, including ways to identify early signs of relapse, they are taught simple (non-emotional) communication skills and problem-solving skills, and are encouraged to expand their social networks.

Compliance therapy/medication management

Stopping medication (sometimes known as **non-compliance**) can be a serious problem in schizophrenia, because someone may need to stay on medication for many years to remain well, and may relapse if it is stopped. However, failing to take the full course of medication is a human failing – how many of us do not finish the entire course of antibiotics we are prescribed? Unfortunately, with mental illnesses, taking all the prescribed medication, every day, may be an essential part of staying well.

non-compliance
Not taking medication as directed. Compliance therapy can be useful to reinforce adherence.

Many people want to stop their antipsychotic medication as soon as possible, and do not realize, or do not accept, that they are likely to become ill again. They will often say things like, 'Well, I didn't take the medication all last week and I feel even better', not realizing that most medication stays in the body for weeks, and stopping for a single week is not likely to make an immediate difference (except for clozapine which only stays active in the body for a few days). People may not understand what a relapse could cost them, or that the illness could be progressive. Relapse is associated with further impairments in social functioning and has an impact on relationships.

Medication is of course associated with risks in terms of side effects, and the inconvenience of taking it. The key to successful treatment is the choice of medication such that side effects are reduced to a minimum, and the person taking the medication is happy to do so.

A number of factors have been shown to help people to stay on their medication. These include:

✧ an acceptance of their illness
✧ an understanding of their susceptibility to relapse
✧ the level of support available
✧ family stability
✧ a positive therapeutic alliance with the prescriber
✧ a simple medication regime.

You can imagine how difficult it could be to remember, for example, to take three different tablets at varying times of the day. In addition, side effects, the failure of the medication to improve symptoms, poor communication between the person taking the medication and the prescriber, and substance abuse are associated with the person stopping their medication.

Compliance therapy is sometimes known as medication management. It uses CBT techniques, information and education to address the factors listed above, engaging with the person taking the medication, exploring areas of ambivalence, providing information about the medication and

compliance
In this case it means to take medication as directed. Also known as 'adherence'. Compliance therapy can be useful for those who have difficulty taking their medication.

the risks and benefits, and getting the person involved with, and taking responsibility for, their treatment. These strategies may seem like common sense as well as good nursing and medical practice. However, the success of formal medication management programmes have yet to be firmly established.

my experience

A case of 'non-compliance': John came for a second opinion because his psychiatrist had tried everything, and John was no better. John came to the clinic on high doses of clozapine, amisulpride, chlorpromazine, an antidepressant, clomipramine and a sleeping tablet. He had been an inpatient for the past ten months with prominent delusions and hallucinations, and he was intermittently violent in response to his voices. Despite this, John retained a sense of humour and social awareness which made his psychiatrist very keen to find the right medication to help him.

John had no side effects whatsoever, despite the large quantities of medication he was taking. We asked him how he coped with all that medication. 'That's easy, doctor,' he replied. 'I just don't take any of it.' John was congratulated on his ability to pull the wool over the eyes of the nurses who handed out his medication (either putting it under his tongue, or up his sleeve, or occasionally even regurgitating it). He responded well to an explanation about medication and what it was designed to do. His fear of side effects (caused by a really bad reaction to a typical antipsychotic early in the course of his illness) was confronted and explanations given, and he eventually agreed to take the clozapine.

John did very well and was discharged to his own flat within six months. He is now prominent in local affairs, belongs to a political party, and is the Chair of the Resident's Association for his block of flats.

Cognitive remediation therapy (CRT)

Cognitive impairment is characterized by a range of problems in a person's thinking abilities. It is an important symptom of schizophrenia which has received less attention than positive and negative symptoms, but which is highly correlated with outcome, and can be a barrier to complete recovery. Any intervention which can improve mental functioning is likely to lead to benefits in living skills and the ability to function independently.

Cognitive remediation therapy is a fairly recent therapy which is not yet widely available. There are a variety of methods, but all are designed to improve thinking skills. First, any specific cognitive problems are identified through testing. Next, exercises of increasing complexity are given to target the specific cognitive problems (usually on a computer, but they can be done with pen and paper) and finally, an evaluation of the intervention is made by giving another round of cognitive testing.

CRT can lead to improvements in social functioning and adjustment and raise self-esteem.

cognitive remediation therapy
Therapy designed to improve thinking skills.

Rehabilitation programmes

The goal of modern treatment is to enable people with schizophrenia to be as functional as possible in society. **Rehabilitation** programmes have a three-pronged approach:

rehabilitation
Refers to the process of recovery, support and reintegration into family/ home / work following illness. With schizophrenia this may take many months and is likely to require professional support.

1 The illness is improved as much as possible with medication and psychotherapy.
2 People are taught social skills, life skills and problem solving techniques.
3 They are housed in a supportive environment that is suitable for their needs and wishes.

Most rehabilitation programmes are centred on a particular hostel or similar facility, where the person remains for a set period of time, usually between one and three years.

Self-management

This is a programme of support and education aimed at helping people to take active steps towards their own recovery. It is usually user-led and user-guided. Individuals are encouraged to take control of their lives, and not to let their condition rule them. For individuals well enough to participate in this programme, self-management can lead to enhanced self-esteem and increased motivation.

Conclusions

✧ Antipsychotic drugs treat psychotic (positive) symptoms. Their effect on the negative symptoms is variable. They can be divided between the older *typical* antipsychotics and the newer *atypical* antipsychotics, with a more complex mode of action, and where side effects may be less of a problem. Clozapine (taken with safeguards) is reserved for peole with schizophrenia which is unresponsive to other medications.

✧ Medication can be taken in a variety of different ways, including pills and injections (known as depot).

✧ All antipsychotics can cause a very wide range of side effects. These include: extra pyramidal side effects (EPSEs, sometimes known as Parkinsonian side effects, which are usually reversible; anticholinergic (muscarinic) side effects; anti-adrenergic side effects; side effects associated with increased prolactin hormone; effects on the heart; weight gain; effects on metabolism and a range of other side effects.

✧ Remember to consult your doctor if you have any worries about side effects as usually these can be managed by a switch to an alternative antipsychotic. Don't just stop taking the medication as this can cause relapse.

✧ Usually a person who has had psychosis should continue their medication for at least one full year after the psychotic symptoms have stopped.

✧ Most people with schizophrenia will be offered an antidepressant at some stage of the illness, because depression frequently accompanies schizophrenia. They can also be offered mood stabilizers to augment the antipsychotic medication, or if mood is a particular problem.

✧ There are non-drug treatments that can also help: cognitive behavioural therapy (CBT) which focuses directly on core psychotic symptoms such as delusions or hallucinations; family therapy which reduces high expressed emotion (High EE) within families; compliance therapy/medication management which encourages people to accept and take their medication. Other helpful interventions include cognitive remediation therapy (CRT); rehabilitation programmes and self-management programmes.

CHAPTER

6 Living with schizophrenia

The key to living with schizophrenia, for both people with the illness and those close to them, is to understand, accept and then learn to manage the illness with the help available.

Early treatment

It is said that there are as many ways of experiencing schizophrenia as there are people who have it. The early stages of a psychosis can be very frightening, and a natural reaction can be to pretend it is not happening, but it is very important to seek help early. Early treatment is seen as so vital that dedicated 'Early Intervention Teams' have been set up to offer treatment as soon as possible (see Chapter 8).

Chapter 2 explored the difficulties of diagnosing schizophrenia. However, psychosis is not difficult to diagnose, and antipsychotic medication helps with psychosis in general, rather than for schizophrenia in particular. The best way forward is usually to treat the psychosis, and worry about the precise diagnosis later.

Concerns for people with schizophrenia

The symptoms of schizophrenia (positive/psychotic, negative, cognitive and depression) can lead to problems in almost every area of life (social, work, interpersonal and the ability to care for yourself in basic ways). Sometimes dealing with these interlocking problems can seem overwhelming (see figure).

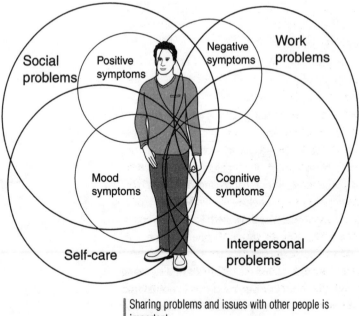

Sharing problems and issues with other people is important.

It is important to accept all the support and help available, whether from people close to you, your doctor, or the mental health team. Sharing problems and issues with other people is important – don't try to deal with it alone.

Physical health

It is a surprising and shocking statistic that people with schizophrenia die, on average, ten years younger than someone without this diagnosis. There are a number of reasons why this might be. Suicide is more common in schizophrenia, and accounts for some deaths, but this is not the whole story. Accidental death is also more common in schizophrenia, and while some apparently accidental deaths may really be suicide, some people with schizophrenia, if they are acutely unwell, may be inattentive to their personal safety. Poverty may be another reason for early death.

People with mental health problems are also more likely to suffer common illnesses. Diabetes is five times as common in people with mental health problems and heart disease and respiratory disease are twice as common. HIV is eight times more likely, and Hepatitis C is 15 times more likely. People with severe schizophrenia may be inattentive to their own physical problems or indicators of ill-health, or their efforts to express their worries may be downplayed. Maggie's story, in Chapter 7, illustrates the case of a woman with severe chronic schizophrenia who developed breast cancer but did not tell anyone, and when the disease was found it was very advanced.

A further cause of early death is associated with the side effects of medication. Too much medication, given without regular monitoring of physical health, can lead to health-threatening side effects. Of course, worries about side effects of medication have to be counterbalanced against the detrimental effects to health of not taking medication at all. The side effects of medication are outlined in Chapter 5. Common problems to watch out for, which may or may not be to do with medication, are diabetes, weight gain and heart disease. These three conditions tend to cluster – obesity can lead to diabetes and heart disease.

From April 2004, GPs have been able to choose to provide more services to people with severe mental illness, under the new GP contract. They can create a register of people with bipolar disorder and schizophrenia, for which they are paid extra money. Most patients would benefit from annual blood pressure checks, a urine test for diabetes, weight monitoring, cervical cytology (women), breast examination (men and women), chest and heart examination and discussion of smoking habits, and a review of medication. Some medication can have an effect on electrical conduction in the heart, and yearly electrocardiograms may be advisable.

It is important that attention is paid to the physical health and lifestyle of anyone with a severe mental disorder. Regular exercise and attention to weight and diet are particularly important.

Smoking

People who are very unwell with chronic schizophrenia and who have a poor outcome are particularly likely to smoke cigarettes. Over 70 per cent of people in hospitals or hostels for the mentally ill smoke, compared to about 25 per cent of the general population. Several reasons have been put forward for this; nicotine could have a beneficial effect on negative schizophrenic symptoms, but the association with severe schizophrenia suggests that this is not the case. Smoking could improve the side effects associated with some antipsychotic medication; it can be shown that smoking stimulates enzymes in the liver which metabolize antipsychotic drugs and so smokers have lower drug levels in the bloodstream than non-smokers. It is also the case that nicotine can stimulate a release of dopamine, and therefore negate some of the adverse effects of dopamine blocking medication. So far, research has not been able to provide any clear answer to these questions. It is particularly important, however, for smokers to have regular health checks.

Substance misuse

We know that using drugs such as cannabis, cocaine, ecstasy, amphetamines and LSD can trigger the first episode of schizophrenia. Drugs can also perpetuate symptoms and lead to relapse. Many people find the immediate effects of the drugs comforting and helpful (particularly cannabis), not realizing that these drugs are worsening any underlying psychosis. Unfortunately, illicit drugs are a problem on most hospital inpatient wards. People with both psychosis and substance misuse problems ('dual diagnosis') are not well supported by the NHS. They are not accepted by most services dedicated for people substance misuse, and most community mental health teams are ill-equipped to deal with such problems.

Pregnancy

There are a number of issues surrounding the decision to have a child, if the mother or father has schizophrenia. First, the person needs to be well enough to handle the disruption and sleep disturbance associated with having a baby in the house. Second, if the parent with schizophrenia is the mother, there may be issues concerning medication during and after pregnancy, and the risk of relapse after the birth has to be taken into account.

If possible, all medication should be avoided in the first three months of pregnancy. However, many people stay on antipsychotic medication throughout pregnancy. Typical antipsychotics have been used in pregnancy for many years and are generally considered to be safe, but there is little information concerning atypical antipsychotics because they have not been available for as long as typical drugs. The decision whether to continue medication during pregnancy should always be taken with your doctor. However, approximately 50 per cent of pregnancies are unplanned, so care should be taken with contraception if the medication is known to be toxic to the unborn baby (for example, lithium or certain anti-epileptic drugs).

Even if the mother and baby are safe and well on a particular antipsychotic throughout the pregnancy, there may be problems of withdrawal for the baby after it is born. For this reason, the mother's medication may be stopped before the birth, but this is not always possible.

After any birth, mood changes occur in 75 per cent of mothers, and these mild mood changes are known as 'baby blues'. Psychosis is rare, and usually means that the mother has a diagnosis of bipolar disorder or schizophrenia. Many doctors recommend starting medication again as soon as possible after delivery, if a mother has a pre-existing psychotic illness.

Then there is the decision about breast-feeding. Medication differs as to whether it is present in breast milk. Typical antipsychotics have been used in breast-feeding mothers for many years and they are considered safe. There is less information about the newer atypical medications, largely because there has been insufficient time for information to build up. Clozapine is contra-indicated because it accumulates in breast milk.

Antidepressants are secreted in breast milk in small quantities, and it is generally safe to continue to take antidepressants while breast-feeding.

Of the mood stabilizers, lithium is secreted in breast milk and is contra-indicated. Carbamazepine and sodium valproate are also found in breast milk but do not appear to have any negative effect on the baby. However, there should be careful consideration of the risks and benefits before either of these is used. There is little information on other mood stabilizers.

Q Is it safe to breastfeed if you are taking medication for schizophrenia?

A Some medication can be safe but not others. Always discuss with your doctor.

Social isolation and poor quality of life

Many people who have had schizophrenia find it difficult to find a place in society once their illness has been treated. Problems such as lack of confidence, poor social skills, stigma against mental illness, and difficulties finding employment can prevent a full recovery. Mental health services are often overstretched and cannot extend provision to those who are not acutely ill, or who have no immediate problems. There is no short answer to these problems. Persistence and determination in asking for help is essential, and by taking little steps forward regularly, a person's quality of life can be greatly improved.

my experience

Omar was an only child; his mother nearly died giving birth to him, and could not have any more children. Despite his difficult birth, Omar did well at school and went on to university in 1981. Unfortunately he had a severe psychotic breakdown at university and was diagnosed with schizoaffective disorder. He was in hospital for six months. Omar was started on a depot antipsychotic which was a great help, and he continued to receive it from a nurse at his GP surgery for the next 25 years, living at home, seeing no one socially and doing little except household chores and visiting the local library. His parents always took care of all the bills and made all the decisions. By 2003 Omar's parents were in their late fifties, and both were unwell. His father had diabetes and had had a heart attack, and his mother had had bowel cancer. They were uneasy about Omar's future and asked for him to see a psychiatrist.

Omar described his problems: 'The medication has been a great help, I think. It has its price, but I'm afraid not to take it; I was so ill. I feel "flattened" and find it difficult to talk to people; I don't know if that's me, or the medication. When I talk to people they look at me strangely, and I think maybe I look different or something. No one wants to have anything to do with me, but perhaps I don't mind that so much. I don't really have anyone but my parents, and if anything happens to them I don't think there will be any reason for me to live on'.

At the clinic, Omar was found to have some side effects of the depot injection, which caused his tongue to twitch, and his hands had a rhythmic tremor at the wrist [these are EPSEs – see Chapter 5]. He was taken off his depot and, after discussion with him and his parents he was given a trial off medication. Omar had been started on the depot injection after his first breakdown. [Most prescribers, nowadays, would recommend stopping the medication one to two years after recovery from a first psychoatic breakdown, if the person remains well.] Omar was encouraged to attend a local community centre and was lucky enough to be allocated a befriender, who encouraged him to get out more and join a book club. Omar has a much more positive view of the future without his parents.

Concerns for carers

Coping with the diagnosis

Sometimes, parents will focus on their worries about the diagnosis and treatment of their child's illness, and fail to get any treatment at all by resisting the diagnosis. They worry about doing the right thing. Rachel's story, below, illustrates what happened to her adopted daughter, Sara.

my experience

Keith and I adopted Sara when she was only a few weeks old. Her birth mother was supposed to be very wild, and Sara was one of three girls. They all had different fathers. We were lucky enough to get Sara and her older sister Carlie, but there was only an 18 month gap in their ages, so it was hard work to begin with! Sara was always slower than Carlie, and slower than other children we knew, and she was always a clumsy girl, but it was nothing major. Sara always wanted to be a good girl. She was a happy child. She did reasonably well at school to begin with, but from the age of 13 she started staying in her room a lot, and did not get any GCSEs.

When she was 17, Sara went with her sister Carlie to spend time on a project doing voluntary work in Africa. Keith and I didn't hear much from them during the six months they were there. When she got home, Sara wanted to get a job, but she said she was worried because she didn't have any qualifications, and she never applied for anything. Months went by. Sara seemed to 'switch off'. Most of the time she kept herself to herself in her room. If I tried to get her to come out she would scream and cry that she had 'lost her thoughts', and kept saying that she wanted to be 'like her old self'. I thought she needed counselling, but when I suggested it to her, Sara just cried and cried. Then one night she insisted that we should call out the doctor. He talked to her for about half an hour, after which the crisis team was called in, and Sara was admitted to hospital – just like that. I still think the doctor over-reacted. It was the wrong thing to do.

Sarah hated it in hospital, and I could not bear to see her in there. All the other patients seemed so 'rough' and Sarah was like a little lost soul. We had to have her home. Maybe it wasn't the right thing. Since then Sarah has been very withdrawn, and she does not appear to understand what people say to her any more. She stays up late watching TV, but I'm not sure she really watches it, it is just on. Then she stays in her room all day. She sometimes says things like 'her thoughts are taken away' or 'her thoughts are gone'. She never says much. But she's never heard voices. I ask her about that all the time. One of the doctors said she had schizophrenia but I don't think that can be right. She's such a quiet gentle little thing unless she goes into one of her rages, and then she screams like a banshee and throws things around. Maybe some therapy to do with her anger would help, but I can't get her to go. Maybe she feels abandoned by her birth mother. They gave her some pills in hospital but they only made her fat and filled her with toxins, so I told her to stop them. I just don't know what to do. She's been like that for two years now.

Sara's problems illustrate the difficulty people can have accepting schizophrenia as a diagnosis, and their search for any other problem that might fit the bill. It also illustrates some of the mistaken ideas people have about schizophrenia; Rachel thought schizophrenia meant hearing voices and because Sara did not hear them, she did not have schizophrenia. Rachel disliked the weight gain Sara had with the medication, and took it upon herself to tell her daughter to stop the tablets, without realizing that this could mean Sara's illness might become worse, if it was untreated.

Rachel and Sara were helped, in the end, by information about schizophrenia, education about negative attitudes and communication patterns, and detailed information about medication. Rachel was put in touch with other parents whose children have schizophrenia, and she was able to share her concerns with them. Sara was started on a medication which does not cause weight gain. It is too early to tell how much she will benefit from this.

Problems of confidentiality

There is sometimes a tension between clinical information about someone with schizophrenia which doctors feel they have to keep private, and that information which families or other people close to someone with schizophrenia feel they need to have in order to offer the best help and support.

Doctors and mental health professionals have an ethical duty to keep patient information confidential. Patients have a right to expect this. There are only a few situations where a mental health professional *has* to disclose information, for example if ordered by the Court, if there is a concern that serious harm may occur to a third party, or if the police are conducting a criminal investigation which would be affected if the information was withheld.

On the other hand, families often feel 'out of the loop' and excluded from information about

confidentiality
Not disclosing information about a patient.

the illness itself, the medication and its side effects, relapse indicators and outcome.

There are historical reasons why psychiatrists might tend to err on the side of withholding information. Chapter 4 outlines the views of the 'anti-psychiatrists' who saw schizophrenia as a result of poor family interaction or poor parenting. Obviously, in that situation, it might be reasonable to keep information about the person with schizophrenia confidential, but we now know that this is not true, and where there are problems in family interactions, they are best addressed by an open discussion, information and advice. However, these old ideas hang on in traditions and teaching, and many families gain the impression (rightly or wrongly) that confidentiality is used as a smokescreen to prevent them from learning anything at all.

Nowadays, we realize that families are in the best position to help if they know as much as possible about the problem. The Royal College of Psychiatrists recognizes this, and encourages the psychiatrist to discuss information sharing with the patient and record their responses in the notes. Consent to disclosing information must be informed (i.e. the person knows what they are consenting to), the person giving the consent must have real choice, and there must be some expression of consent verbally or in writing. However, the psychiatrist is free to, and should, discuss the benefits of sharing information with the person's family, and also the benefits of obtaining information from the family. In an initial interview, some people feel more comfortable if their family are spoken to first so that nothing they have said to the psychiatrist can be revealed, or they may opt to have a family member present during the interview. If a person refuses consent for information sharing, then the psychiatrist can arrange for the family to be given general information about the illness which does not reveal anything about the individual in question.

Eamonn was brought for a second opinion by his parents, who felt certain he had a diagnosis of schizophrenia, but their problem was frustration over his lack of progress, and reluctance on the part of their local mental health team to make any diagnosis. Eammon's story, below, is told by a junior doctor in a psychiatric clinic.

my experience

Eamonn is 32 years old, and lives with his parents. His parents brought him to the clinic because he is doing nothing at all in life, and they are sure he has schizophrenia. Eamonn does not tell them anything about his illness, although he sees a psychiatrist. On this occasion, Eamonn was willing to come to the clinic with his parents, and said he did not mind if the doctors spoke to them.

Eamonn's parents were seen first. They say that the first time they knew of any mental health problems was when Eamonn was asked to leave college, when he was 19 years old. When he came home, he was behaving strangely, lying in bed surrounded by candles, which he said were there to 'protect himself'. He was sleeping poorly and not eating. Eamonn was seen by a psychiatrist at home, and after that he was taken on by the local clinic and prescribed medication, but was never given a diagnosis. Eamonn's parents say he did not take his medication, and after that 'nothing seemed to happen' for many years until he had to be **sectioned** into hospital five years ago because he was not eating and had not left his room for several weeks. He was diagnosed with an acute schizophreniform psychosis on this admission, and was prescribed depot antipsychotic medication, which has been given by the community nurse ever since. Eamonn's parents feel 'out of the loop'. They have been told that Eamonn is a grown man, and his therapy is a private matter which Eamonn does not wish to share with them.

sectioned
To be involuntarily detained in hospital under one of the 'sections' of the Mental Health Act 1983.

When Eamonn himself was interviewed, he adopted an amused and 'lofty' manner. At times, during the interview, Eamonn laughed for no apparent reason, or frowned, or muttered to himself. Eamonn said he had no psychiatric problems at all. When asked about his family, and whether he was able to talk to them about his illness, he said, 'My parents are called smokey dragons and I would love to talk about communication with them but they are like lizards.' During the interview, Eamonn appeared disinterested in the conversation, often staring into different corners of the room as if there was something there, or out of the window. He said his thoughts were controlled by the 'souls of demons and reptiles' who were his 'role models'. He said the demons told him how to behave, and when they were angry with him they would pin him to his bed, but he said he 'tries to accommodate them as much as possible' and he can usually leave his room for short periods. After being interviewed for about ten minutes Eamonn left the room abruptly and went and sat in the waiting room.

Eamonn's parents were informed that it was not possible for us to discuss what Eamonn had said with them, but we were writing to the treating team with recommendations, which included a switch to clozapine.

Eamonn's parents were right that he had schizophrenia, and right to be worried about his treatment and lack of progress. As the people closest to him, Eamonn's parents were in the best position to know how things were at home, and they had valuable information to pass on to the treating team. Although Eamonn had a right to confidentiality, it was not in his best interests for his parents to be excluded from decisions about his care.

After this clinic visit, Eamonn was persuaded to accept another admission to hospital, where he was started on clozapine. After several months Eamonn began to improve and he was discharged home. He was seen again two years later, when the contrast with his original visit was remarkable. Eamonn was still living at home, but he had been able to find a part-time cleaning job in a furniture factory run by a family friend. He was planning to learn to drive and, although he still had a poor social life, he had begun to go to family gatherings and he went to the pub with his dad once a week.

my experience

Jen and Tim were desperate to help their son Jason, who had mental health problems. Jason's problems started when he was in his late twenties. Before then he had been able to start up his own taxi firm and had a girlfriend, and a young son of his own. Jason lost his business due to problems with income tax, and his girlfriend left him. He returned home, but before long he was admitted to psychiatric hospital under a section of the Mental Health Act, after going to his girlfriend's house in the night and breaking her windows. Jason was discharged to his parents' home after ten days in hospital. His parents were not informed of his diagnosis, nor the treatment being offered, and despite trying to contact the psychiatrist and members of the treating team on several occasions, they were never given an appointment.

Jason was willing to come for a second opinion, and willing for his parents to be interviewed about him. They had never had a chance to talk to anyone about their worries and concerns before, and were very willing for information they gave to be given, in turn, to Jason. When he came to talk about his problems, Jason admitted to feelings of anger towards his parents whom he felt had not been sufficiently helpful when he lost his business, and also shame that he had been unwell and admitted to mental hospital. He was astonished that they were so worried about him, as he perceived them as uncaring.

Several weeks later Jason's parents wrote to say that the opportunity for them to voice their concerns had been helpful in itself, but they were also able to have an open discussion with Jason, which had cleared the air, and he had told them about his problems in more detail, including his diagnosis (acute psychotic episode).

What is illness and what isn't?

Many people don't understand or accept that people with schizophrenia cannot control their behaviour or symptoms. It is perhaps easier to accept that positive or psychotic symptoms cannot be controlled. However, negative symptoms of lack of motivation can seem very like laziness, and altered emotions or lack of emotion can mistakenly be equated with lack of love. Most people who are close to someone with schizophrenia on a day-to-day basis will benefit from an opportunity to talk over the person's symptoms with a professional, perhaps a member of the Community Health Team, or with another relative in a similar situation.

What to say to someone who is deluded or hallucinating

It is important not to minimize or dismiss such symptoms, or try to argue the person out of them by pointing out the illogicality of what they are saying. It is best to respect what the person is saying or experiencing, without colluding with it: for example, 'I understand that you believe that people are talking about you and that someone is plotting against you. That must be very frightening for you, and I can understand and sympathize, although we must agree to differ about whether it is true.' There are educational programmes (mentioned in Chapter 4) where carers can learn to understand and manage the illness.

Drug abuse and blame

Substance misuse is increasingly recognized as a risk factor for schizophrenia. People with the illness can sometimes feel guilty and remorseful – 'if only' they had never used drugs, while their loved ones can feel angry, and see the illness as 'his/her own fault'. Both attitudes are as unhelpful as blaming a cigarette smoker when they get lung cancer, or someone who is overweight for eating too much. Where is the person who has never made a mistake in their lives? Ideas about blame and fault can prevent people from moving forward into the phase of acceptance and recovery, and need to be discussed and worked through.

Conclusions

◇ Seek help early.
◇ Try to understand, accept and then learn to manage the illness with the help available.
◇ Watch out for physical health problems.
◇ Pregnancy and bringing up a baby is a possibility for someone with schizophrenia, but there may be difficulties, and the decision should be taken with professional advice.
◇ Problems of confidentiality cannot be a bar to carers receiving general information and advice about schizophrenia.
◇ Carers should avoid blaming people with schizophrenia for their symptoms (no, they are not lazy) or their behavioural problems, including problems with illicit drugs.

CHAPTER

7

How mental health services developed and the problems we face today

The historical context of services for people with schizophrenia, particularly the development of **community care**, can be helpful in understanding the complexity of current services, the current gaps in provision, and future plans.

The old asylums

Up to 50 years ago, care of people with schizophrenia was centred on large mental hospitals ('asylums', a word originally meaning 'sanctuaries'). These were mostly built in Victorian times and were situated on the outskirts of towns, where there was fresh air and a green environment (most Victorian cities being dirty smoky places with high rates of infection). These asylums filled rapidly throughout the end of the nineteenth and early twentieth centuries, reaching a peak occupancy of around 140,000 in the 1950s. We have seen in Chapter 4 how standards fell and a spirit of pessimism grew in these large asylums. The Mental Health Acts of the day were not conducive to the rights of people with mental illnesses, and many people, sometimes unnecessarily, lived out their whole lives in these institutions. They were known as 'long stay' patients (see 'My experience'– Maggie's story).

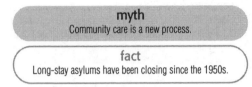

myth
Community care is a new process.

fact
Long-stay asylums have been closing since the 1950s.

From the 1950s to the present day, all but a tiny number of long-stay beds closed, although the number of beds used for acute admissions to hospital (and the needs for these beds) remained constant. In part this change arose because of the success of antipsychotic medication (see Chapter 5), and in part because it was felt to be a better thing, and more socially inclusive, to treat people with chronic mental health problems in the community rather than hidden away in big asylums. There were also hopes that closing the big asylums would lead to cost savings, but this did not prove to be the case.

my experience

Maggie's story: Maggie was born in 1947, the daughter of a doctor, and became ill with schizophrenia in 1962 when she was just 16 years old. There was effective medication available at that time and this was offered to Maggie, but unfortunately Maggie's illness did not respond and she became more and more unwell. By the age of 18 she had effectively become a long-stay patient in a big mental hospital in the countryside outside a major city. Maggie suffered with auditory and visual hallucinations and prominent delusions, and her illness was complicated by violent thoughts towards other people. Her parents remained regular visitors, but Maggie was often violent towards them, and she also assaulted other patients, sometimes with knives or sharp scissors. She was detained as an involuntary patient under the Mental Health Act from the 1960s onwards and the periods when she was allowed out on leave became less and less frequent. Her last overnight visit home was in 1973.

Up to the 1990s, the big asylum where Maggie was detained was a bustling place, with many other long-stay patients who became a kind of family for Maggie. She enjoyed photographing the other inmates, and had a relatively settled life on a women-only ward. There was a hospital shop and regular 'dances' with the men from the male wards. Then the decision was taken to close the hospital. All the patients were assessed for transfer to a community placement, but Maggie was never well enough to move, although she was assessed on several occasions. The big hospital gradually closed, until Maggie was in one of two remaining wards which formed part of a designated secure unit [see Chapter 8 for an explanation of these]. Maggie was with younger patients, many of whom had committed criminal offences and who required specialist secure placements, and for a time she was on a mixed-sex ward, for the first time in her life. Maggie was very distressed by these changes and the loss of her 'community', and her illness worsened considerably.

In 2000 the old asylum closed completely and Maggie was moved to a secure unit within an inner city hospital. There she was given, for the first time, the antipsychotic medication, clozapine, and she was for a time remarkably improved. After several months she was discharged to a 'half-way house'. Unfortunately, a policy of the house at the time was that residents were allowed to administer their own medication. Although Maggie agreed to take the clozapine, in practice she did not do so, and she quickly relapsed. She became so unwell that it was never possible to get her to agree to take clozapine again, and soon afterwards she was found to have advanced breast cancer, for which she refused all treatment. Maggie must have had symptoms for some time, but she had told no one. Her doctors felt that her reasons for refusing treatment were rational, and Maggie died, aged 53.

Community-based care

By the mid-1990s, the transfer of care of people with chronic mental illness from hospital to the community was well under way, but there were many teething troubles with these new services. GPs were neither trained nor prepared for their new role as a linchpin of service provision for the mentally ill, and were unsure what was expected of them. The community was not 'ready' and was prejudiced against the influx of people with chronic mental health problems, and the people with those chronic problems were often too ill, or lacked sufficient motivation, to actively engage in the services which were provided. There was a lack of resources – tragically the money released by closure of the asylums was not reinvested in community services, which remained the responsibility of the local authorities – and the inpatient provision remaining was underestimated, particularly in inner cities, where the incidence of severe mental disorders could be up to nine times that found in some rural areas. At the peak of the problem, in the mid- to late-1990s, there were some inner city psychiatric hospital wards with 140 per cent bed occupancy (only possible because some patients were out on leave). Lack of inpatient beds still remains a problem.

People with serious and chronic mental health problems usually required attention from both health services and social services. However, in the 1990s, health and social services were entirely separate organizations, with different remits and responsibilities and, most importantly, separate funding. This led to 'tussles' about who would pay for ongoing care, people sometimes being 'trapped' in hospital because social services would not agree to take over their care. Other people found themselves 'forgotten' by one service or another.

Maggie's story illustrates the difficulties some people faced when the big old asylums closed. Fortunately, few people were as ill as Maggie, but most did find moving on very hard indeed, at least to begin with. The teething troubles with the new community services were such that some people floundered without adequate care, and their lives were impoverished for a time, rather than enhanced by the move to the community. Community services have proved to be, if anything, more expensive than the old asylum system, and funding was often not in place, so that some people languished in bedsit accommodation without anything to do during the day. Most of these problems have now been addressed, and it is recognized that the quality of life of people with long-term illnesses has been improved by community care. It is important to point out, also, that fears about violence in the community have not been realized. Some people were afraid that, once mental patients were housed in hostels on ordinary streets, rather than in asylums away from everyone else, there would be an increase in violent behaviour and homicide. This has not proved to be the case. However, there continues to be local resistance or 'nimbyism' (not in my back yard) to the establishment of hostels or other mental health facilities, in many areas.

Currently, while some problems have been resolved now that health and social services are organized together, there remains some fragmentation within mental health services because of the number of different new teams being introduced. This can lead to lack of communication, where one team, such as the Crisis Team, does not have access to information held by the Community Mental Health Team. There are also the continuing problems in attempting to deal with people who are acutely ill and suicidal in the community, where there may be insufficient resources for round-the-clock supervision. There have been problems, too, with the over-optimistic closure of beds, leaving some services with too few. This can lead to people being discharged too early, in order to free up beds.

Since the 1990s, government (Conservative and Labour) have provided a series of legal frameworks or statutory advice for mental health, beginning with the NHS and Community Care Act and the **Care Programme Approach** in 1990. These are described in Chapter 8. In 1999 the National Service Framework was set out (see below) and in 2002 the National Institute of Clinical Excellence issued guidance for the treatment of schizophrenia (see Chapter 5).

Care Programme Approach
A long-standing system (since 1990) for people with mental health problems who need care and support from mental health services.

Mental health is currently seen as one of the three biggest health priorities, alongside cardiac care and cancer.

The National Service Framework (NSF) for Mental Health, 1999

This is not statutory, or enforceable, but advisory. It lays down models of treatment and care which people with mental illness, and their carers, are entitled to expect.

The NSF is organized into seven 'standards' for provision of care, which are set in five main areas.

Standard 1 suggests that health and social services should promote mental health issues, educate and disseminate information and combat discrimination and stigma. *Standards 2 and 3* cover GP (primary) care and general access to mental health services, including the standard that mental health needs should be identified and assessed, effective treatments offered, and referral on to specialist services provided. The availability of round-the-clock local services is an identified standard.

Standards 4 and 5 cover services for people with a severe mental illness, and cover topics such as the Care Programme Approach and aftercare as outlined in Chapter 8. It includes the standard that everyone with a severe mental illness should have timely access to an appropriate hospital bed or alternative.

People were delighted to see the needs of those caring for people with severe mental illness recognized in the NSF. *Standard 6* suggests that carers should have a yearly assessment of their caring, physical and mental health needs, and their own written care plan.

The final standard, *Standard 7*, concerns the prevention of suicide. It is suggested that local health and social care agencies should prevent suicide by implementing the other standards, supporting local prison staff, ensuring that staff are competent to assess suicide risk, and conducting suicide audits to learn lessons and take any necessary action. Unfortunately, there is little evidence that there are, as yet, any measures which can reliably prevent suicide.

While there are no statutory rights involved in the National Service Framework, it is helpful for people to see what the government believes to be the appropriate guiding values and principles, and it has contributed to a general improvement in the services offered. It was particularly helpful for many carers to see that they were recognized, even if they had no absolute 'right' to expect Standard 6 to be implemented.

Mental health, social exclusion and employment

Being 'in work' has important implications for well-being. Work brings in money, of course, but also other benefits. It can enhance social identity, provide support and social contacts, provide a strong framework for day-to-day life, and, not least, provide a sense of personal achievement. People who are unemployed for six months are more than three times as likely as others to report the symptoms of depression. Unemployment seems to heighten anxiety and reactivity to stress. It is well known that people with mental illness are particularly sensitive to the negative effects of unemployment and the loss of the positive benefits which are associated with work.

Currently, only 24 per cent of adults with mental health problems are in work, despite disability discrimination legislation. The government's social exclusion unit has recently reported on ways to help people with mental health problems enter and retain work, although it must be recognized that people with schizophrenia may have a degree of disability that makes work unlikely, and pressure to undergo assessments may be poorly tolerated. There are other problems. Many people with schizophrenia, who are comparatively well, risk significant reduction in their benefits (and therefore their sense of security and quality of life) if they venture into work, and the job breaks down. Rules concerning work and benefits remain a big disincentive to trying to work. Some people conclude that it just isn't worth the risk.

However, on the plus side, there are employers who are immensely supportive of people with disabilities. The 'Pathways to Work' initiative, set up to get people with schizophrenia back to work has had some success, and Job Centre Plus has dedicated teams to work with people with disabilities. Sadly, the complexity of the current benefit rules tends to undermine these positive steps.

Conclusions

◇ Today, most people with schizophrenia are treated in the community rather than in mental hospitals.

◇ Problems remain with the delivery of community services.

◇ Government initiatives such as the National Service Framework have been helpful by laying down models of treatment, including carer support.

◇ Some form of employment is an important and often achievable goal for people with schizophrenia.

CHAPTER

8 Services for people with schizophrenia

There have been tremendous changes in the provision of care for people with schizophrenia over the past 50 years, as described in Chapter 7. Social care for those with day-to-day problems in caring for themselves, and psychiatric care providing support and treatment are nowadays almost amalgamated and usually work together. Services are organized on a geographical basis, often incorporating specific GP surgeries. Unfortunately the kind of service available around the UK is not uniform, and there may be local difficulties with lack of personnel or funding. There is also a general lack of choice; in most cases there is only one possible mental health provision available, and only one possible consultant psychiatrist.

It is important to note that most people who have mental health problems are not in contact with mental health services. Although 15 per cent of people in the community are experiencing a significant mental health problem at any given time, only about two per cent will consult a mental health professional.

The first steps

It is important to seek help as early as possible for any mental health worries. It is increasingly recognized that the earlier schizophrenia is treated, the better the outcome is likely to be. Many people, if they worry or suspect that they, or their loved one, has a serious problem, have a tendency to 'wait and see' and hope the problem resolves itself in time. If the problem is schizophrenia, then that can be the worst thing to do. Many people do not like the idea of medication, but effective medication, explained fully, and given in the early stages of the illness, can

⟡ lead to much less medication being required over a person's lifetime
⟡ reduce the risk that the illness will progress to chronic disability
⟡ reduce the need for admission to hospital.

In addition, early treatment minimizes the length of time that someone spends away from their usual activities and lifestyle, makes it easier for them to resume normal life when the illness is under control, and causes less of a strain on family relationships.

It is always important to remember that schizophrenia is a very variable illness in terms of severity and recovery, and in some cases can be very mild indeed. Even if you think you, or someone you are close to, falls into the 'very

Q I'm worried about my teenage son's behaviour. He has changed and has become very withdrawn and unsociable. Should I contact the doctor or wait to see if it's just a teenage phase?

A Seek help as soon as possible. Early treatment for schizophrenia can lessen the impact of the illness and lead to a better outcome.

mild' category it remains important to seek help and information early on.

The GP

The first person to contact if you, or someone you care for, has worries about their mental health, is your GP. If the GP thinks it necessary, he or she will organize an assessment by the local Community Mental Health Team (CMHT), which cares for people with serious mental disorder in a defined geographical area. This can usually be arranged on an emergency basis. GPs are not required to refer someone on to the local CMHT just because they ask for a referral, and sometimes a GP will have sufficient training, or feel confident enough, to treat a mild early psychosis in the surgery. The GP remains ultimately responsible for the care of their patients.

There are sometimes problems when a GP feels unable to accept information from a family about a relative who seems to be developing mental illness. This may be because of misunderstandings about patient confidentiality. In this situation, advice can be sought from Rethink or NHS Direct, or sometimes another GP in the practice is more at ease with mental health problems.

Hospital: Accident & Emergency

Sometimes things reach a crisis without there being the time, or opportunity, to see the GP. If someone goes to A & E with a mental health problem they will be seen by a junior doctor, the psychiatrist on call, or specialized nurse, and access to one of the services described below should be arranged, if necessary.

Mental health services for outpatients

The Community Mental Health Team (CMHT)

The CMHT has been the backbone of mental health services for over 20 years. It is usually composed of a consultant psychiatrist, mental health nurses, occupational therapist and administrator, and may also have assigned social workers and **psychologists**. There may also be junior doctors at various stages of their training. SHOs (senior house officers) are in their second year after medical school, and are in the first stages of becoming a psychiatrist. SpRs (specialist registrars) who have their psychiatry qualification, may also be members of the team. The CMHT may also contain support workers.

GP referrals to the CMHT are assigned to a given professional within the team to interview and arrange for ongoing care. Sometimes this is the doctor, sometimes a CPN (community psychiatric nurse), social worker or occupational therapist. Interviews can take place at the CMHT's headquarters (in hospital or a community centre), or in the person's own home.

After the interview, a decision will be taken at a CMHT meeting about what (if any) service to offer. For some problems associated with schizophrenia, there could be a course such as anxiety or anger management, or medication, medical or CPN support. Other treatments are occasionally available, such as cognitive

psychologist
A general term for a person who studies the mind. Covers a wide range of disparate disciplines. Generally not a qualified doctor.

behavioural therapy (CBT) which may be tailored specifically for psychosis or depression. CMHTs do not have to offer a service if they do not feel the person needs it, they can refer the person back to the GP with appropriate advice.

However, the individual may be designated as being in need of specific services for the mentally ill (under the Care Programme Approach – see below), or in need of a hospital admission.

Where a service is offered, contact with the CMHT may be time-limited, so that the person is referred back to their GP once treatment has been put in place. CMHTs in different parts of the country are not uniform in terms of their composition or what they can offer. If there are difficulties with funding, or recruitment, or if the CMHT is in a particularly needy part of the country, they may restrict the care they offer to individuals with the most severe problems.

Early Intervention Teams

Early intervention services are a recent introduction to the NHS, and came about because of the recognition that the earlier any psychosis, but particularly schizophrenia, is treated the better the outcome will be. Early Intervention Teams normally cater for individuals aged between 14 to 35 who are experiencing their first episode of psychosis and/or are in the first three years of their illness. The teams aim to reduce delays in diagnosis and treatment, and thereby reduce the disruption that can be caused by a psychotic illness. Every individual entered into the service is allocated a key worker, who becomes the first port of call for any problems, and also an agreed Care Plan which covers any other mental health problems, or substance misuse. The team also deals with all the building blocks of every day living, such as housing, finances, physical health, education and employment and family support. The Early Intervention Team will liaise with other services if the person needs hospital admission. The composition of the team is similar to the CMHT described above, and may consist of psychiatrists, nurses, occupational therapists, social workers support workers and administrators. Access to the team is generally via the GP, or a hospital Accident and Emergency.

my experience

Dan's story: I started smoking at school. We all did, if you didn't smoke, at my school, you were a bit pathetic. We smoked spliffs. We'd go to my mate's house, where everyone was out all the time, and sit in my mate's room and smoke. If my mate's mum smelt anything when she came in, she never said. She was okay. We'd smoke the spliff, or we'd use a bong. [Note: a method of smoking cannabis through water in an upside down plastic soft drinks bottle to make the 'hit' stronger.] We drank a lot of alcohol too, if we could get it. We had some good times. I dunno when it happened, but I'd start to get really frightened and 'antsy' all the time. A spliff helped, but then I'd get wary and paranoid. I thought my mum and her partner were watching me and making a tape of my life. I couldn't talk to them about it – that was part of the plan, or something. Actually, I never have told them about it. I just smoked more and it seemed to help. At school, it got so that I couldn't sit anywhere but at the back – if anyone walked behind me, I was gone. Then I couldn't go out at all – everyone was talking about me, and it all seemed planned, or something. One of my mates kept coming round for me, but then he stopped. My mum was a pain. She'd try to talk to me, but I just wanted to be left alone to sleep or whatever. I'd go out to get the stuff, but that was it. It seemed the easiest way to handle it. My mum got the doctor out, but I couldn't talk to her, and then Tony (a nurse with the Early Intervention Team) came. It was all about stopping smoking spliffs and that, and there was medication, but it was a help.

Dan was able to describe his psychosis quite well. Many people are not able to talk about things so freely, or cannot find the words. Dan was quite lucky because his GP was able to call in professional help from the Early Intervention Team at a very early stage, and Dan's **paranoia** responded to low dose antipsychotic medication. Dan continued to smoke spliffs, although much less than before, but the medication (olanzapine) seemed to prevent the paranoia and anxiety. After a time, with the help of his keyworker, Dan was able to stop using cannabis, and he went to college, where he found a girlfriend, and made other new friends. He stayed on the olanzapine for two years, but then felt able to stop it. At the time of writing, Dan is at art college and remains well.

> **paranoia**
> A state in which an individual suffers from a sense of persecution and unwarranted suspicions.

Services for people with ongoing mental health needs

The needs of most people with a milder illness can be covered by contact with the CMHT, where the psychiatrist may prescribe medication, and/or a community psychiatric nurse may provide ongoing support and talking treatments. However, someone may be ill enough to be designated as being in need of services based on a care plan or programme.

Case management: The Care Programme Approach, Care management and Section 117 aftercare

There are three overlapping systems which provide a framework for the ongoing care of people with mental illness living in the community:

◇ **Care management** is provided by social services, and provides for people who need care and support in the community, who may or may not have had specialist psychiatric help.

◇ **The Care Programme Approach (CPA)** is a longstanding system (since 1990) for people with mental health problems who need care and support from mental health services, and is provided by health and social services together.

◇ **Section 117 aftercare** is for people who have been detained treatment sections of the Mental Health Act (for example, sections 3 and 37).

Care management, the Care Programme Approach and Section 117 aftercare are effectively integrated as health and social services now work together, usually via the CMHT. Discussions about these generally occur at the regular CMHT review meetings, where all the professionals on the team meet up to discuss the people under their care.

There are four main stages to the CPA:

1 A co-ordinated assessment of the person's health and social care needs.

2 The development of a Care Plan which will be agreed by an identified care coordinator (who may be any member of the social care/medical team and the patient if possible) and any carers involved.

3 The Care-Coordinator (Key Worker) will be the main contact and will monitor the Care Plan.

4 There will be regular reviews of the Care Plan.

There are two levels of complexity of the CPA, standard and enhanced, depending on the needs of the person in question.

Alternatives to hospital

Crisis Resolution/Intervention Teams

Crisis intervention was highlighted as a need in the National Service Framework (1999) described in the previous chapter. The aim is to respond to and support adults with severe mental health problems who might need admission to hospital, and to manage and resolve the crisis at home, without hospital admission becoming necessary. (Hospital admission remains available, however, if the crisis cannot be resolved at home.) A good Crisis Intervention Team can reduce the need for hospital admission by a third.

These teams may be organized differently and can have different names, such as home-based crisis services, home treatment services or acute home treatment. Out-of-hours services, rapid response services, crisis services and psychiatric emergency services may be slightly different, but fulfil the same function. The Crisis Intervention Service and the Early Intervention Service may be one and the same. The composition of the team is similar to the CMHT described earlier, and may consist of psychiatrists, nurses, occupational therapists, social workers support workers and administrators.

Crisis resolution/intervention should offer flexible, home-based care, seven days a week. Their response is rapid (sometimes within the hour) and interventions are generally short-term, perhaps up to a month. If need be, the service will then refer the person on to another service for ongoing care or hospital admission. Access to the team is usually via the GP, a hospital emergency room, or another mental health team.

Assertive Outreach (Community Treatment) Teams

This is a newly developing service which works with people who have severe and lasting mental illness who cannot or will not engage with traditional services. The caseloads are generally smaller than in the CMHTs. The team members work with the person in their own environment, in a flexible manner, forging a trusting, longer-term relationship. They can help with all the problems of everyday living, and help to build trust between the person and the health service. A good Assertive Outreach Team can reduce the need for hospital admission, reduce the length of hospital admissions, and reduce the need for admission under the Mental Health Act.

Community centres (day centres)

Most people have access to community centres which offer a drop-in service, allowing people non-pressured social contact, as well as various courses and therapies. However, many of these are being closed, on the basis that services specifically designed for the mentally ill are stigmatizing. However, there is a worry that the needs of people with severe and chronic problems may be ignored.

Day hospitals

In the past, most aftercare took place in the hospital setting. Many people were admitted to 'day hospitals' if they were felt in need of an intensive programme of care, but could remain at home. Most day hospitals have closed or are closing, and their functions have been taken over by community centres. Again, there are worries about the needs of people with severe and chronic problems.

Residential facilities

People who cannot live independently can be offered supported accommodation. This may vary from the simple provision of hostel accommodation, to hostels where staff call in, up to those offering round the clock support. This may form part of a rehabilitation programme, in which case the individual is expected to move on after a number of years, or be a home for life. There is currently a shortage of accommodation for people who have a high level of need and most supported accommodation (other than care homes) is now funded under the 'Supporting People' scheme, which requires people to move on within two years, to a more independent living situation.

Benefits for people with mental health problems

People with mental health problems may be able to claim for accommodation, prescriptions, home help, travel and other costs. There is a wide variety of benefits available. People with mental health problems may be able to claim a basic income benefit, help with rent and extra benefit to cope with their needs to support their daily living. There are also benefits for those returning to work, and benefits for carers.

The benefits system is very complex. If you have a mental health problem you may not feel up to making a claim, and you may get into debt, which may make matters worse. Very many people miss out on what they are entitled to claim, and their lives are less comfortable, and their mental illness can be worse, as a result. Even if they know that they should claim, the forms can be difficult to fill in. If you have a serious mental health problem, and you have been assigned a Care-Coordinator, then he or she may help you to apply. The Department of Work and Pensions itself will help with filling out forms etc. by phone. When in doubt contact your local Citizens Advice or the Rethink National Advice Service.

Admission to hospital

An individual with mental health problems may be very unwell when first seen by their GP, or when they attend the hospital A & E department. A visit by a consultant psychiatrist, the CMHT or one of the other teams described above may be organized as an emergency, but sometimes admission to hospital is felt to be the best way forward. Some people, who have been admitted to hospital in the past, find that it is helpful to have time away from everyday pressures and they actively seek an admission.

Admission to hospital can be on a voluntary or involuntary basis. Voluntary admissions are the majority, and take place on exactly the same basis as admissions for a physical illness. The person is free to go when they wish to do so, and does not have to accept the treatment offered.

Formal, or involuntary admission refers to admission under the Mental Health Act (1983). About 15 per cent of hospital admissions occur in this way. This may be necessary if the person lacks insight into their illness and resists treatment.

There are a variety of hospital wards available. The most usual is the open ward, where patients are free to move about as they wish. Most hospitals also contain one or more locked wards, which are used if the person is at particular risk of harming themselves or others, or if their mental health is felt to warrant involuntary treatment which the person is unwilling to accept. 'Locked' wards may not be actually locked, but the person is prevented from leaving by nursing staff. Locked wards are sometimes known as acute wards or high dependency wards. Individuals who have chronic mental health problems, who are ready to leave the acute ward or the open ward, but who are not ready to return to life outside the hospital, may be transferred to a rehabilitation ward where there are specialist staff who work with the person to get them back into everyday life.

Compulsory admission to hospital

The Mental Health Act (MHA) (1983) covers the assessment, treatment and rights of people with a mental health disorder. It allows people with a mental disorder to be detained (usually in hospital) and given treatment without their permission. This Act will be amended but remains in force at the time of writing. Individuals may be assessed for compulsory admission in their own homes, in a hospital A & E, or when they are already admitted to an open ward.

Section 2 of the Mental Health Act

Section 2 refers to admission for up to 28 days for assessment and treatment and cannot be renewed, but it can be converted to Section 3 – see below.

The **approved social worker** (ASW) and two doctors believe that:

1 The person has a mental disorder of a nature or degree which requires them to be detained in hospital for assessment or assessment and treatment.
2 The person needs to be detained in hospital in the interests of their health, personal safety, or to protect other people.

> ### approved social workers (ASW)
> A qualified social worker in the mental health field who has been trained to carry our designated functions, including making an application for detention in hospital under The Mental Health Act 1983.

Section 3 of the Mental Health Act – Reasons for hospital admission

Section 3 refers to admission for up to six months and can be renewed. Detention is for a specific form of mental disorder such as mental illness. The mental disorder should be of a nature or degree that means the treatment should be given in hospital. The person needs treatment for their health or safety, or to protect other people, and this treatment can only be given if the person is detained under Section 3.

Section 4 of the Mental Health Act – Admission for assessment in cases of emergency

This is used for someone who needs to be detained in hospital urgently and there is insufficient time for them to be seen by a second doctor. The ASW remains involved as before. The person can be detained in hospital for up to 72 hours on the recommendation of a single doctor, once a second doctor has examined the person, and if that doctor agrees, the section changes to Section 2.

fact
You can also be admitted under section on the grounds of
health.

If circumstances change, and the mentally ill
person agrees to remain as a voluntary patient, or
their illness improves sufficiently so that they no
longer need to be detained in hospital, then the
responsible doctor (**RMO** or Responsible Medical
Officer – usually the consultant psychiatrist) must
rescind the Section.

RMO
Responsible Medical
Officer – the formal
term for the
psychiatrist in charge
of a patient's care
when detained in
hospital under The
Mental Health Act
1983.

fact
A doctor can bring the section to an end at any time.

Who decides if it is appropriate to use the MHA (1983)?

The decision must be made by two doctors and
a third person, who must all agree that an
admission under the MHA is necessary. One of
the doctors must have special experience with
mental disorders and, if possible, one of the
doctors should know the person. The third
person is usually an approved social worker
(ASW) who has specialist training and experience
in dealing with people with a mental disorder. A
close relative (called the **nearest relative**) can
also apply for a person to be detained, but this
rarely happens.

nearest relative
An appointment made
by The Mental Health
Act 1983 according to
a list set out in the Act.
The nearest relative
has legal rights in
respect of a person
involuntarily detained
in hospital. Not
necessarily the same
as the next of kin.

Q Who is the 'nearest relative' under the MHA (1983)?

A The nearest relative is formally defined, and cannot be chosen. Determining who is the nearest relative is very complex and there is a formula in the MHA which determines who has the role (usually a close relative). This person does not have to accept 'nearest relative' responsibility, and can give it up or assign it to someone else.

The rights of the nearest relative

The nearest relative can apply for the mentally ill person to be admitted to hospital. The local authority has a duty to consider compulsory admission, usually by the ASW interviewing the person, if the nearest relative requests it. The nearest relative must be told if an ASW applies for the person to be detained. The nearest relative can object to the application for detention, but the ASW can ask the Court to appoint someone else as nearest relative if the ASW thinks the objection is unreasonable. The nearest relative can also apply for the person to be discharged from hospital, although the doctor in charge of the case can stop this.

The rights of the individual detained under the MHA (1983)

The hospital itself should write informing the person what section they are detained under, what it means, and the right to apply to a Mental Health Review Tribunal to have the section lifted. The individual is also given information about how and when treatment can be given without consent, why the person is being detained, and information about the Mental Health Act Commission (which visits hospitals where people are detained and checks that their detention is lawful).

The Mental Health Review Tribunal (MHRT)

This is a statutory, independent, body which is responsible for hearing the appeals of patients who are detained in hospital under the MHA.

Each individual tribunal consists of three people; a legal person (the Chair), a psychiatrist, and a lay member who usually has mental health experience. The patient, their doctor, and their social worker are seen by the tribunal. The tribunal can recommend discharge, leave of absence, supervised discharge, conditional discharge or transfer to another hospital, and they can adjourn or reconvene as necessary. Anyone who appeals to a MHRT is entitled to legal representation. (There is also a separate form of appeal to the Hospital Managers.)

Proposals to amend the Mental Health Act (1983)

There are plans to amend the current Mental Health Act, which will come into force in 2008. This decision by government followed seven years preparation for new mental health legislation, which has eventually been dropped. The 2008 amendment will bring the 1983 Act up to date and ensure its compatibility with human rights law. A more modern and wider definition of mental disorder is proposed, and there will also be the introduction of compulsory treatment orders for some people living in the community. There will also be a new right for people in contact with the mental health services (whether or not detained) to apply to the County Court for their nearest relative to be displaced, either if the relationship is damaging to their health and well being or if it has broken down altogether. The role of the approved social worker will be replaced by that of the approved mental health professional and is to be opened up to others, perhaps nurses or psychologists. Some of the changes discussed over the years, such as advance statements, advocacy, care plans and sharing information with carers will be introduced in a new Code of Practice.

Special hospitals and secure units

These hospitals and units are designed for the small number of patients who are at very high risk of harming themselves or others. Direct admissions to such hospitals are possible, but most patients will have come from a general mental health facility, or through the Courts because of involvement in criminal activities. Individuals admitted to a special hospital must present a significant danger to the public and require the highest level of security. Secure units offer a lower level of security and are used for people who are too disruptive for an ordinary hospital. They are normally on specialized Sections of the Mental Health Act.

Forensic psychiatric teams

There is a special branch of psychiatry dedicated to the needs of patients who are, or have been, in special hospitals, secure units or prison, or people who have become involved with the police or the Courts. This is known as 'forensic psychiatry'. Psychiatrists specializing in forensic psychiatry substitute general training for two to four years specialist training.

It is a well-known and unresolved problem that many people with mental illness are in prison rather than in a psychiatric hospital. These people are overwhelmingly young men who have psychiatric and substance misuse problems which have led them into trouble with the law.

Conclusion

Seek help early – do not be frightened

The care systems outlined in this chapter can seem complicated and daunting. It may be frightening to read about the Mental Health Act and compulsory admission when you have only minor worries about your own or someone else's mental health. You may worry that if you go to the GP and are diagnosed with schizophrenia you could end up in hospital against your will when you have no need to be there. In practice, services are strictly tailored to a person's needs and there are very firm checks to prevent anyone being admitted to hospital who does not need the admission.

The need to seek help as early as possible is so important that it bears repetition. Early intervention leads to a better outcome and reduced need for medication and hospital stays.

Interested

Afterword

Seeking help is an essential first stage in dealing with the distress and worry of a developing mental disorder. Problems which seem terrifying and insurmountable alone can often be solved with the right help. It is important to remember that many other people have experienced similar difficulties before, and found solutions to their problems. There is a wealth of experience and information available both in the NHS and through voluntary organizations. Hopefully the information in this book will be a useful guide.

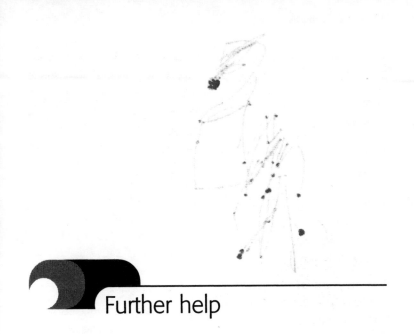

Further help

Below is a list of support organizations. The list is not exhaustive but links to other organizations should be available from those listed below.

Bipolar Fellowship Scotland
(formerly Manic Depression
Fellowship, Scotland)
Mile End Mill
Studio 1016
Seedhill Road
Paisley PA1 1TJ
Tel: 0141 560 2050
(Helpline)
Fax: 0141 560 2170
email: info@bipolarscotland.org.uk
web: www.bipolarscotland.org.uk

Helps people with bipolar disorder/
manic depression and their carers
throughout Scotland.

Carers UK
Ruth Pitter House
20/25 Glasshouse Yard
London EC1A 4JT
Tel: 020 7490 8818
Fax: 020 7490 8824
email: info@ukcarers.org
web: www.careruk.org
Hours of opening: Mon–Fri
9.00 a.m.–5.00 p.m.
Carer's line: 0808 808 7777

Carers UK is a campaigning
organization providing information
and advice on all aspects of caring
to both carers and professionals.

Carer's line is a free advice line for carers.

Hafal
Suite C2
William Knox House
Britannic Way
Llandarcy
Neath SA10 6EL
Tel: 01792 816 600
Fax: 01792 813 056
email: hafal@hafal.org
web: www.hafal.org

Support organization in Wales for those with severe mental illness and their carers.

HCC (Health Care Commission)
London Head Office
Finsbury Tower
103–5 Bunhill Row
London EC1Y 8T9
Tel: 020 7448 9200

The Health Care Commission promotes improvement in the quality of the NHS and independent healthcare.

JAMI (Jewish Association for the Mentally Ill)
16A North End Road
London NW11 7PH
Tel: 020 8458 2223
Fax: 020 8458 1117
email info@jamiuk.org
web: www.jamiuk.org

Jewish charity offering services and support to sufferers from severe mental illness, their carers and families.

Together (Formerly Mental After Care Association, MACA)
First Floor
Lincoln House
296–302 High Holborn
London WC1V 7JH
Tel: 020 7061 3400
Fax: 020 7061 3401
email: contactus@together-uk.org
web: www.together-uk.org

Together is a leading mental health charity providing community services including advocacy, assertive outreach schemes, community support, employment schemes, forensic services, information, respite for carers, social clubs and supported accommodation.

MDF The Bipolar Organisation
Castle Works
21 St Georges Road
London SE1 6ES
Tel: 08456 340 540 (UK only)
Tel: 0044 207 793 2600 (rest of the world)
Fax: 020 7793 2639
email: mdf@mdf.org.uk
web: www.mdf.org.uk

User led charity working to enable people affected by bipolar disorder/manic depression to take control of their lives.

MDF The Bipolar Organisation Cymru
22–9 Mill Street
Newport
South Wales NP20 5HA
Tel: 01633 244 244
(Helpline: 08456 340 080)
Fax: 01633 244 111
email: info@mdfwales.org.uk
web: www.mdfwales.org.uk

Supporting those with bipolar disorder/manic depression in Wales.

Mental Health Act Commission
56 Hounds Gate
Maid Marian House
Nottingham NG1 6BG
Tel: 0115 943 7100
Fax: 0115 943 7101
email: chiefexec@mhac.org.uk
web: www.mhac.org.uk

The main role of the commission is to keep under review the operation of The Mental Health Act as it relates to the detention of patients.

Mental Health Foundation, The
9th Floor
Sea Containers House
20 Upper Ground
London SE1 9QB
Tel: 020 780 1100
Fax: 020 7803 1111
email: mhf@mhf.org.uk
web: www.Mentalhealth.org.uk

A major UK charity for those with mental health problems or learning disabilities. It promotes research, service development and the communication of information to increase understanding and meet people's needs.

Mental Health Foundation (Scotland)
5th Floor
Merchants House
30 George Square
Glasgow G2 1EG
Tel: 0141 572 0125
Fax: 0141 572 0246
email: scotland@mhf.org.uk
web: www.mentalhealth.org.uk

Similar role in Scotland to MHF above.

Mental Health Matters
Avalon House
St Catherines Court
Sunderland Enterprise Park
Sunderland
Tel: 0191 516 3500
Fax: 0191 549 7298
web: www.mentalhealthmatters.com

Working in partnership with service users and their families, friends and health professionals to maximize the quality of services.

Mind (The National Association for Mental Health)

Granta House
15–19 Broadway
London E15 4BQ

Mind infoline: 0845 766 0163
Tel: 020 8519 2122
Fax: 020 8522 1725
email: contact@mind.org.uk
web: www.mind.org.uk

Leading mental health charity, providing a national information and legal service as well as local groups offering a range of support services. Campaigns for a better life for those diagnosed as mentally ill and their right to lead an active and valued life in the community.

Mind Cymru

3rd Floor, Quebec House
Castlebridge
Cowbridge Road East
Cardiff CF11 9AB
Tel: 029 2039 5123 (office only)
Fax: 029 2034 6585

A leading mental health charity in Wales, working to ensure that people who experience mental health distress, their carers and friends, are treated with respect, given equal access to services and opportunities in the community, and do not have their rights abused.

NHS Direct (England and Wales)

Operates a 24-hour health information service.
Tel: 0845 46 47
web: www.nhsdirect.nhs.uk
web: www.nhsdirect.wales.nhs.uk
(for Wales)

NHS24 (Scotland)

Operates a 24-hour health information service in Scotland
Tel: 08454 24 24 24
web: www.nhs24.com

National Institute for Mental Health in England

Room 8E 46
Quarry House
Quarry Hill
Leeds LS2 7UE
Tel: 0113 254 5127
email: ask@nimhe.org.uk
web: www.nimhe.org.uk

Supporting positive change in mental health services.

Northern Ireland Association for Mental Health

Central Office
80 University Street
Belfast B17 1HE
Tel: 028 9032 8474
email: edassistant@niamh.co.uk
web: www.niamh.co.uk

Provides local support for those with mental health neeeds across Northern Ireland.

Richmond Fellowship
80 Holloway Road
London N7 8JG
Tel: 020 7697 3300
Fax: 020 7697 3301
web: www.richmondfellowship.
org.uk

Helps people with mental health problems to live and recover in services that are designed to restore an individual's sense of security, purpose and fulfilment. Has community mental health services including registered homes, supported housing, back-to-work schemes and outreach teams.

Royal College of Psychiatrists, The
17 Belgrave Square
London SW1X 8PG
Tel: 020 7235 2351
Fax: 020 7245 1231
email: rcpsych@rcpsych.ac.uk
web: www.rcpsych.ac.uk

Professional and educational organization for psychiatrists in the UK and Republic of Ireland. It produces user friendly materials for the general public on common mental health problems and treatments.

Sainsbury Centre for Mental Health, The
134–8 Borough High Street
London SE1 1LB
Tel: 020 7827 8300
Fax: 020 7403 9482

email: contact@scmh.org.uk
web: www.scmh.org.uk
Hours of opening: Mon–Fri
9.00 a.m.–5.00 p.m.

The Centre aims to improve mental health services through a co-ordinated programme of research, service evaluation, service development and training.

Samaritans, The
For support, write to:
Chris
PO Box 9090
Stirling SK8 2SA
Helpline: 08457 90 90 90 (UK) &
1850 60 90 90 (Ireland)
Office tel: 020 8394 8300
Also has local branches, details in phone book or operator can put you through.
Fax: 020 8394 8301
email: jo@samaritans.org
web: www.samaritans.org

Offers confidential emotional support 24 hours a day to those in crisis and in danger of taking their own lives.

SANE
First Floor
Cityside House
40 Adler Street
London E1 1EE

SANELINE: 0845 767 8000 (calls charged at local rates)

Tel: 020 7375 1002
Fax: 020 7375 2162
email (admin only):
london@sane.org.uk
web: www.sane.org.uk

SANE seeks to change attitudes about mental illness, campaigning for improved rights and care and conducting research through the SANE research centre. Runs Saneline, a national mental health helpline.

Scottish Association for Mental Health (SAMH)
Cumbrae House
15 Carlton Court
Glasgow G5 9JP
Tel: 0141 568 7000
email: enquire@samh.org.uk
web: www.samh.org.uk
Hours of opening: 9.00 a.m.–5.00 p.m.

A leading independent voluntary organization concerned with mental health in Scotland.

Making Space
46 Allen Street
Warrington
Cheshire WA2 7JB
Tel: 01925 571680
Fax: 01925 231402
web: www.makingspace.co.uk

Helps people affected by the problem of schizophrenia and other forms of enduring mental illness in the North of England. It provides support advice and help to people in their own homes through locally based Family Support Workers.

National Schizophrenia Fellowship (Scotland)
Claremont House
130 East Claremont Street
Edinburgh EH7 4LB
Tel: 0131 557 8969
Helpline: 01224 213 034 for Grampian region
Fax: 0131 557 8968
email: info@nsfscot.org.uk
web: www.nsfscot.org.uk

Offers advice, information and support to people who have experienced mental illness, their families and carers. Support groups for carers meet throughout the country and the services include a range of drop-in/resources centres and employment training schemes.

RETHINK (Formerly The National Schizophrenia Fellowship)
Head Office
5th Floor
Royal London House
22–5 Finsbury Square
London EC2A 1DX

Rethink
Registered Office
28 Castle Street
Kingston-Upon-Thames

Surrey KT1 1SS
Tel: (general enquiries) 0845 456 0455
National Advice Service: 020 8974 6814
Fax: 020 7330 9102
email (general):info@rethink.org.uk;
email (for advice): advice@rethink.org
web: www.rethink.org

The leading national mental health membership charity, works to help everyone affected by severe mental illness recover a better quality of life. Their aim is to make a practical and positive difference by providing hope and empowerment through effective services and support, including mutual support groups, for those who need it. Rethink believes that those who experience severe mental illness are entitled to be treated with respect and as equal citizens, and actively campaigns for change through greater awareness and understanding.

RETHINK (Northern Ireland)

(Formerly the National Schizophrenia Fellowship)
Regional Office
Wyndhurst
Knockbracken Health Care Park
Saintfield Road
Belfast BT8 8BH
Tel: 028 9040 2323
Fax: 028 9040 1616

email: info@nireland.rethink.org.uk
web: www.rethink.org

RETHINK (Northern Ireland) exists to help people with severe mental illness, their families and carers. The services provided are: flexible day care centres province-wide, supported accommodation, flexible employment service, training and employment services and information and advice.

Hearing Voices Network (HVN)

79 Lever Street
Manchester M1 1FL
Enquiries and information
Tel: 0845 122 8641
Helpline: 0845 122 8642
email: info@hearing-voices.org
web: www.hearing-voices.org

HVN is a network of voice hearers, allies, mental health professionals and other interested parties and has a network of self-help groups throughout the UK. It offers information about voice hearing, disseminate research and help in setting up groups.

Schizophrenia Ireland (also called the Lucia Foundation)

Head office
38 Blessington Street
Dublin 7
Ireland

Tel: +353 (0)1 8601620
Fax: +353 (0)1 8601602
Helpline: +353 (0)1 890621631
email: info@sirl.ie
web: www.sirl.ie
National organization in Republic of Ireland addressing needs of those with schizophrenia and related illnesses.

Threshold Women's Initiative
National free phone for women experiencing mental health difficulties and/or emotional distress and their carers.
Helpline: 08088 086000 (Calls answered by women.)

Turning Point
A social care organisation providing services for those with complex needs, including those affected by drug and alcohol misuse, mental health problems and those with a learning disability.
Tel: 020 7702 2300
web: www.turning-point.co.uk

UKPPG National Mental Health Drugs
Helpline: 020 7919 299 (available 11 a.m–5 p.m. weekdays)
Provides free independent advice and information about mental health drugs.

Glossary

The glossary contains terms that you may hear being used about schizophrenia as well as a number of key terms that are used in the book. Some common medical words are often misunderstood (e.g. 'chronic'); others (e.g. 'compliant') are used in a specialized way in psychiatry.

Acute (of illness)	Serious, and arising quickly.
Aetiology (American English 'etiology')	The cause of an illness.
Affect (noun)	Mood (the adjective is 'affective', as in bipolar affective disorder).
Akathisia	A feeling of physical restlessness; the person finds it difficult to stay still. A possible side effect of antipsychotic medication.
Anti-adrenergic side effects	Possible side effects of antipsychotic medication; can include a drop in blood pressure when standing up suddenly (postural hypotension), and a range of sexual problems such as inhibition of ejaculation.

Anticholinergic (muscarinic) side effects	Possible side effects of antipsychotic medications on the muscarinic receptors (can include rapid heart rate, dry mouth, constipation, difficulty urinating, blurred vision).
Antidepressant (medication)	Major classes include the tricyclics, the selective serotonin re-uptake inhibitors (SSRIs), and the monoamine oxidase inhibitors (MAOIs).
Antipsychotic (medication)	Drugs used to treat psychosis, divided into typicals (older drugs) and atypicals (more recent drugs with different side-effect profile). Pamphlets on medication can be obtained from Rethink.
Antisocial personality disorder	Personality disorder diagnosed when an individual has psychopathic traits (often criminal) and the absence of remorse. (Note antisocial in this context does not mean 'bolshie' but is used in a much stronger sense, meaning persistently against society.)
Assertive Outreach (Community Treatment) Teams	A newly developing service which works with people who have severe and lasting mental illness who cannot or will not engage with traditional services.
Assessment	An evaluation of an individual's mental state and needs. There are also special forms of assessment, such as Risk Assessment.
Avoidant personality disorder	Characterized by low self-esteem, social awkwardness, and fear of being viewed negatively by others.
ASW (Approved Social Worker)	A qualified social worker in the mental health field who has been trained to carry out designated functions, including making an Application for detention in hospital under the Mental Health Act 1983.
Bipolar disorder	A mood disorder in which an individual alternates between the two 'poles' of (1) depression and (2) the overexcited state of mania. Also known as bipolar affective disorder, and manic depression.

Borderline personality disorder	Characterized by a pattern of unstable personal relationships, uncontrolled anger, fear of abandonment, impulsive/manipulative behaviour, problems with mood and self-image. Often accompanied by frequent self-harming and/or suicide threats. More common in women. Psychotic features can be confused with schizophrenia.
Cannabis	Illegal street drug. Using cannabis in early adolescence can lead to a four-fold increase in risk of developing schizophrenia.
Care Program Approach (CPA)	A long-standing system (since 1990) for people with mental health problems who need care and support from mental health services.
Care-Coordinator	The named mental health professional with overall responisibility for co-ordinating and monitoring the care plan and who will generally have the most contact with a patient in the community.
Care Plan	Plan drawn up, following assessment, by mental health professionals together with the patient and, ideally, with his/her carers, which sets out a plan for the patient's treatment and support.
Catatonic stupor	Rare complication of schizophrenia or bipolar disorder in which the individual becomes completely motionless, does not speak or eat and is unable to look after himself. Catatonic schizophrenia is a sub-type of schizophrenia, though rarely diagnosed.
Chronic (of illness)	Of long duration and recurrent; may be mild in degree. Often mistakenly thought to mean 'serious'.
Clusters	Groupings; personality disorders are arranged by DSM-IV-TR into three clusters: Cluster A (paranoid, schizoid, schizotypal); Cluster B (antisocial, borderline, histrionic, narcissistic);

	Cluster C (avoidant, dependent, obsessive-compulsive). There is often considerable overlap within each cluster, and the diagnosing of personality disorders is far from an exact science.
Clinical	Often used in psychiatry to mean 'psychiatrically significant', hence 'clinical depression', which means depression which needs medical attention, as distinct from the everyday 'blues' which everyone may experience.
Clozapine	An antipsychotic for treatment-resistant schizophrenia. Requires ongoing blood testing for risk of neutropenia.
CMHT	*See* **Community Mental Health Team.**
Cognitive	Related to thinking (in all its aspects).
Cognitive behavioural therapy	Use of cognitive and behavioural techniques to change behaviours, attitudes and negative ways of thinking (e.g. 'I'll always fail'; 'I'll always be rejected') with strategies designed to encourage suitable behaviour and positive ways of thinking, thereby boosting self-esteem. A form of cognitive therapy can be helpful in schizophrenia to help individuals cope with and control psychotic symptoms.
Cognitive remediation therapy	Designed to improve thinking skills. Exercises of increasing complexity are given to target the specific cognitive problems.
Compliance (adjective, 'compliant')	Taking medication as directed. Also known as 'adherence'. A special kind of therapy, compliance therapy, can be useful for those who have difficulty taking their medication.
Community Care	A general term for looking after patients in the community (rather than in hospital); now underpinned by a range of legislation.
Community Mental Health Team (CMHT)	Multidisciplinary team which cares for people with serious mental disorders in a defined geographical area.

Confidentiality	Not disclosing information about a patient. There is sometimes a tension between clinical information about someone with schizophrenia which doctors feel they have to keep private, and that information which families or other people close to someone with schizophrenia feel they need.
CT	Computed tomography: a scanning technique that can show brain abnormalities/variations. Uses X-ray source, unlike MRI.
Delusion	A *false* belief which is firmly held.
Dependent personality disorder	Such individuals are excessively 'clinging' and are characterized by a fear of separation, and a desire to be taken care of.
Depot medication	Slow-release medication given by injection.
Disorganized schizophrenia	*See* **hebephrenic schizophrenia.**
Dopamine	A neurotransmitter. It is thought that overactivity in the dopamine systems is implicated in the generation of psychotic symptoms in schizophrenia. Antipsychotic drugs work, in part, by blocking dopamine.
Double bind	An outdated and wrong idea that parents induced mental illness in their offspring by repeatedly placing them in intolerable situations.
DSM-IV-TR	American Psychiatric Association Diagnostic and Statistical Manual of Mental Disorders, Fourth Edition, Text Revision. Washington, DC, American Psychiatric Association, 2000. Together with ICD-10, one of the two standard psychiatric texts on classification of disorders.
Dual diagnosis	In psychiatry this means substance abuse (usually street drugs and/or alcohol) in addition to a diagnosis of another psychiatric disorder.
Dystonic	Muscles become fixed in abnormal attitudes. A possible side effect of antipsychotic medication.

ECT (electroconvulsive therapy)	A brief, controlled electrical current is administered to the brain for which the patient is anaesthetized and given a muscle relaxant. Can be helpful and a life-saver for very severe depression; now rarely used in schizophrenia.
EPSEs (extrapyramidal side effects)	Side effects of particularly the older typical of antipsychotic medication. Can include movement problems such as tremors, restlessness, muscle spasms, and a shuffling gait as well as a wide range of other problems. Also seen to a lesser extent with some newer atypical drugs.
Eugenics	An outdated and totally wrong idea that the human gene pool could be cleaned up by removing faulty genes. Such ideas were widespread across Europe but, most significantly, were taken up by the Nazi party in Germany before the Second World War.
Family therapy	A therapy designed to alter negative attitudes, expectations and communication within a family where there is a psychiatrically ill member. Can be very useful in reducing problems with 'high expressed emotion'.
Florid (of symptoms)	Strongly in evidence, and not hidden. Usually applied to psychotic symptoms.
Forensic psychiatrist	A psychiatrist specializing in patients who have committed criminal offences.
ICD-10	The ICD-10 Classification of Mental and Behavioural Disorders, Clinical Descriptions and Guidelines. Geneva: WHO, 1992. Together with DSM-IV-TR, one of the standard psychiatric texts on classification of disorders.
Genetic counselling	Counselling about the risk to a family member of the occurrence of a genetic disorder (or partly genetic disorder, such as schizophrenia). This can address many different concerns: 'My son has schizophrenia. How likely are his

children to have it?'; 'I am thinking of adopting a child whose mother had schizophrenia. How likely is the child also to suffer from the disorder?'

Hallucination	False sensory experience with no basis in reality. Senses involved can include one or more of the following: auditory (most commonly, hearing voices), visual, taste, smell or touch.
Hebephrenic Schizophrenia	A sub-type of schizophrenia (also known as 'disorganized'). A form of chronic schizophrenia principally characterized by foolish mannerisms, senseless laughter and delusions.
Heritability	Degree to which a disorder is inherited.
High expressed emotion	(Also known as high EE) It is thought that 'high EE' within families is associated with poor self-esteem, depression and rejection of the diagnosis by family members.
Hippocampus	Part of the brain; thought possibly to be implicated in schizophrenia.
Histrionic personality disorder	Characterized by inappropriate attention seeking and excessive emotional instability.
Hyper-	When used at the beginning of a word means 'excess' or 'over', e.g. 'hyperactivity'.
Hypo-	When used at the beginning of a word means, 'less than' or 'under', e.g. 'hypomanic'.
Hypomanic	Less than full mania but exhibiting some of the symptoms. (Often misunderstood and mistakenly thought to mean 'super' manic.)
Insight (of mental illness)	Refers to an individual's capacity to recognize that he/she is mentally unwell.
Involuntary patient	(Sometimes 'formal' patient) Refers to a person who is compulsorily detained in hospital under the Mental Health Act 1983.
Involuntary movement	Bodily movement not initiated by the person and which may even occur without their knowledge. May result from side effects of antipsychotic drugs.

Labile (of mood)	Subject to rapid change.
Limbic system	Area of the brain involved in sensation and emotion. When the connections in the limbic area of the brain are faulty, errors develop in the ability to process information about the outside world and about ourselves, and this is known as 'psychosis'.
MAOIs	The monoamine oxidase inhibitors – one the major classes of antidepressants, not used as often as tricyclics and SSRIs.
Mania	A condition of over-excitement associated with hyperactivity and sleeplessness, and sometimes grandiosity. Colloquially known as 'high' (although this 'high' has nothing to do with the 'high' from illegal drugs). It is the opposite of depression and is one of the two 'poles' that makes up bipolar disorder (also known as bipolar affective disorder, or manic depression).
Manic depression	An older term for bipolar disorder, though still used.
Mendelian inheritance pattern	Straightforward pattern of inheritance, unlike that found in schizophrenia.
Mental Health Act 1983	The Act which currently sets out the procedures and safeguards for treating and detaining those with mental illness in hospital. In the process of being substantially amended (2006), particularly as regards community treatments.
Mental Health Review Tribunal (MHRT)	A statutory, independent, body which is responsible for hearing the appeals of patients who are detained in hospital under the MHA.
MRI	Magnetic resonance imaging – a brain imaging technique able to detect variation in brain structure; safe for patients to be scanned regularly (unless they have pacemakers or metal plates).
Multiple personality	A rare condition in which an individual takes on one or more additional personalities (Dr Jekyll

and Mr Hyde). Thought to be a variant of severe borderline personality disorder. Not to be confused with schizophrenia.

Muscarinic	(*See* **anticholinergic**)
NSF	National Schizophrenia Fellowship (now known as Rethink). NSF can also refer to the government initiative 'National Service Framework'.
Narcissistic personality disorder	Characterized by an excessive need for admiration, together with fantasy and grandiosity.
National Service Framework for Mental Health, 1999 (NSF)	Government initiative which lays down models of treatment and care which people with mental illness, and their carers, are entitled to expect.
Nearest relative	An appointment made by Mental Health Act 1983 according to a list set out in the Act. The nearest relative has legal rights in respect of a person involuntarily detained in hospital. The nearest relative need not necessarily be the same as the next of kin.
Negative symptoms	One of the two major grouping of symptoms in schizophrenia (the other is 'positive symptoms'). So-called because they represent features that are lost by the person. Negative symptoms include problems with motivation, energy and drive, as well as the ability to think and plan. Negative symptoms are often not understood and may be mistaken for laziness/lack of get up and go.
Neurotic disorders	Disorders that are related to an emotional state, anxiety, depression, or obsession, which though distressing, do not prevent the individual from thinking rationally and functionally socially. Often contrasted with psychotic disorders (such as schizophrenia).
Neuroleptic drugs	Drugs which have an effect on brain functioning.

Neurotransmitter	A chemical messenger in the brain.
Neutropenia	A condition in which there is a reduced number of neutrophils in white blood count. Can be a consequence of drug treatment, particularly, but not exclusively, clozapine/Clozaril/Denzapine/Zaponex. It is a requirement of taking clozapine/Clozaril/Denzapine/Zaponex that ongoing testing for this is undertaken.
NICE	National Institute of Clinical Excellence – produces clinical guidelines, including one covering the medication recommended for schizophrenia.
Non-compliance (Adjective: 'non-compliant')	Not taking medication as directed. Also known as non-adherence. Compliance therapy can be useful to reinforce adherence.
Obsessive compulsive personality disorder	Characterized by inflexible perfectionism, and a wish to control.
Occupational Therapy	Occupational therapy is about much more than hobbies. It teaches skills involving personal care, daily activities, social skills, health care and diet, all of which can greatly assist a person recovering from serious mental illness to regain their independence.
Organic (when applied to mental disorder)	Caused by obvious physical illness, injury or damage.
Panic attack	Sudden attack of fear or anxiety associated with symptoms such as accelerated heart rate, trembling, sweating, shortness of breath, and dizziness.
Paranoia	A state in which an individual suffers from a sense of persecution and unwarranted suspicions.
Paranoid personality disorder	Characterized by an unreasonable suspiciousness of others. This disorder may be wholly unrelated to schizophrenia.
Paranoid schizophrenia	A form of schizophrenia characterized by fixed (often persecutory) delusions, commonly with

auditory hallucinations. Personality is often well-preserved and the condition generally responds well to antipsychotic drugs. It is sometimes wrongly thought by the public that this is the worst kind of schizophrenia and that everyone with this diagnosis is always a danger to others.

Paraphrenia Sometimes used to describe a form of schizophrenia which starts late in life, and which is characterized by delusions but relatively intact personality.

Parkinsonian side effects Side effects of antipsychotic medication that involve abnormal movements, stiffness or tremor. (*See also* **EPSEs**.)

Pathological Related to illness or disorder. In psychiatry often means 'of clinical significance'.

Personality disorder Characterized by inflexible and enduring behaviour patterns that impair social functioning. Some personality disorders, particularly borderline personality disorder can have some similarity to schizophrenia.

PET Positron emission tomography – brain imaging which can investigate the functioning of the brain three-dimensionally. Entails the injection of drugs which are traceable radioactively.

Polypharmacy In the treatment of schizophrenia, this refers to the prescribing of multiple antipsychotics; generally to be avoided.

Positive symptoms One of the two major grouping of symptoms found in schizophrenia (the other being 'negative symptoms'). Positive symptoms are the psychotic symptoms where the normal senses (hearing, vision, touch, smell, taste) may appear faulty due to a failure of the brain to distinguish its own internal activity from things happening in the outside world. Positive symptoms are usual obvious and relatively easy

	to diagnose, compared with the negative symptoms which may be less apparent.
Premorbid	Preceding the onset of illness.
Prodrome (Adjective: 'prodromal')	A period before emergence of illness, where there are early warning signs of problems to come. Before the emergence of schizophrenia there may a gradual social withdrawal/ awkwardness before the diagnosis becomes apparent. Unfortunately it is often only with the benefit of hindsight that this can be recognized. In some cases, there are no such early warning signs and the illness appears suddenly.
Prolactin	A naturally occurring hormone in men and women involved in normal sexual functioning and pregnancy. Some antipsychotics can lead to a rise in this hormone, resulting in a range of sexual side effects.
Prognosis	The prediction of future course of a disorder.
Psychiatrist	A medically qualified doctor who, following training, specializes in the treatment of mental illness and abnormal behaviour. There are four grades of hospital psychiatrists; SHOs (Senior House Officers – a junior grade undergoing training as psychiatrists), SpRs (Specialist Registrars – psychiatrists undergoing higher training), Associate Specialist (fully qualified psychiatrists); Consultant psychiatrists (who lead the team).
Psychologist	A general term for a person who studies the mind. Covers a wide range of disparate disciplines. Generally not a qualified medical doctor. Clinical psychologists, though again not qualified medical doctors, have a specialist clinical training and will often work in hospitals as part of the team.
Psychogenic	Caused psychologically rather than physically.
Psychopath(ic)	Describes an individual with persistent

Psychosis
(Plural: 'psychoses';
adjective: 'psychotic')

antisocial behaviour (often criminal) and the absence of remorse. Also known as sociopath(ic). The formal personality disorder is generally known as antisocial personality disorder.

A mental disorder involving the individual in extreme distortions of thought which lead to a lack of contact with reality. The individual will often have no insight into this process. Schizophrenia is classified as one of the psychotic disorders.

Psychotherapy

There are a wide range of psychotherapies, all of which broadly depend on the patient talking about their problems (and their origins) with the therapist. Can be unhelpful in schizophrenia as the patient requires insight into their illness to engage fully. Some kinds of psychotherapy (for instance, psychoanalytic psychotherapies) can make a patient with schizophrenia worse; others, particularly cognitive therapy, can be helpful.

Psychotic

The adjective from psychosis (*see above*). This is a technical psychiatric term and does not mean 'dangerous' as is commonly thought.

Refractory
(of a disorder)

Fails to respond to treatment.

Rehabilitation

Refers to the process of recovery, support and reintegration into family/home/work following illness. After an episode of schizophrenia this may take many months and is likely to require professional support.

Relapse

Re-emergence of illness. Relapse in schizophrenia can be minimized with appropriate medication and it is almost always important to continue with medication even after symptoms have subsided.

Rethink

Leading charity for those with serious mental illness, including schizophrenia.

Residual schizophrenia	One of the sub-types of schizophrenia. Some symptoms (often only negative symptoms) persist but not in an active phase.
Risk assessment	An assessment of a patient's possible future problems, particularly with regard to the risks of self-harm, harm to others, and relapse. A risk assessment is routine, and having one does not mean that the individual is thought to be at a particularly high risk.
RMO (Responsible Medical Officer)	The formal term for the psychiatrist in charge of a patient's care when detained in hospital under the Mental Health Act 1983.
Schizoaffective disorder	A disorder in which a mixture of schizophrenic and affective (mood) symptoms are displayed. There is a debate in psychiatry about whether this is really a separate disorder. The term is sometimes used when there is diagnostic uncertainty as to whether the primary diagnosis is one of schizophrenia or bipolar disorder.
Schizoid	A personality characteristic of an individual who is solitary and withdrawn. This may amount to a personality disorder (schizoid personality disorder) but it is not the adjective from schizophrenia (which is 'schizophrenic') and 'schizoid' can be diagnosed in individuals who do not have schizophrenia.
Schizophrenia	A psychiatrically defined mental disorder characterized by positive (psychotic) and negative (motivational) symptoms, generally treated with antipsychotic medication.
Schizophrenic	The adjective from schizophrenia (*see above*). This is a technical psychiatric term and should not be used loosely to mean a split personality. This is wrong and unhelpful.
Schizophrenogenic	Causing schizophrenia. A term used in expressions such as 'schizophrenogenic mother', an old and discredited idea of the

anti-psychiatrists that the way a mother brings up a child can cause schizophrenia. Upbringing does not cause schizophrenia.

Schizotypal personality disorder
A personality disorder in which there are some characteristics associated with schizophrenia but without the psychotic symptoms.

Sectioned
To be involuntarily detained in hospital under one of the 'Sections' of the Mental Health Act 1983. Frequently used by mental health professionals, this is not a technical term, although it is widely understood.

Self-management
A programme of support and education aimed at helping people to take active steps towards their own recovery.

Serious mental illness
A term covering the more serious mental disorders, including schizophrenia, bipolar disorder and depression.

Serotonin
A neurotransmitter (known as 5-HT$_2$) and thought to be involved in psychosis. Some medication works by inhibiting the re-uptake of serotonin.

Service User
A term often used by mental health professionals to refer to an individual who is accessing mental health services. Most doctors continue to refer to those they treat as 'patients', as this is a term which emphasises the personal and therapeutic nature of the relationship.

SPECT
Single photon emission computed tomography. Brain imaging technique which can investigate the functioning of the brain three-dimensionally. Entails the injection of drugs which are traceable radioactively.

SSRIs
Serotonin-specific re-uptake inhibitors – one of the major classes of antidepressant medications. Includes Prozac (fluoxetine).

Stigma
Unreasonable and unjustified prejudice within society, caused by ignorance and fear. Those

with schizophrenia often have to bear this heavy extra burden.

Sub-types of schizophrenia
The subtypes of schizophrenia are paranoid, disorganized or hebephrenic, catatonic, and residual. These terms are used less and less and have little bearing on outcome or treatment. The diagnosis of schizophrenia is much more significant than the precise subtype.

Susceptibility
In genetics, having a raised risk on account of genetic make-up. In schizophrenia, having such a raised genetic risk does not mean that a person will inevitably get the disorder. Other non-genetic risk factors will also be important.

Syndrome
A recognized pattern of symptoms. In psychiatry the term (for instance, 'schizophrenia syndrome') is sometimes loosely used to describe a symptom picture which falls short of the full disorder or which is uncertain diagnostically).

Tardive Dyskinesia
A side effect of antipsychotic medication in which the individual has involuntary repetitive movements of the limbs, trunk and face; associated with the older 'typical' antipsychotics.

Temporal lobes
Part of the brain – thought to be involved in schizophrenia.

Therapeutic (Adjective from 'therapy')
Often used in psychiatry to mean 'effective', hence a 'therapeutic dose' of medication is one which is at the right level for the individual patient.

Thought disorder
Present when there are marked abnormalities in the form and flow of thought.

Treatment resistance
Despite compliance, patient fails to respond to prescribed medication. In schizophrenia, clozapine/Clozaril is then generally indicated (subject to safeguards and testing).

Tricyclics	One of the major classes of antidepressants, so classified because of their structure.
Ventricles	Areas in the brain containing cerebrospinal fluid.
Violence in schizophrenia	Exaggerated by the media. Those with schizophrenia are overwhelmingly more likely to harm themselves than others.
Voluntary patient	(Also known as 'informal' patient) A person who is staying in a psychiatric hospital willingly and is free to leave. It is possible for a patient's status to change to 'involuntary' detention while in hospital.
Weight gain	Can be a possible side effect of a wide range of medication taken for schizophrenia. This can be helped with active management.
Working diagnosis	A diagnosis which is not fully determined, but one which forms the basis of treatment. It is relatively common for diagnosis to change in the early stages of a psychotic illness, as often the diagnosis only becomes clear over time.

Index

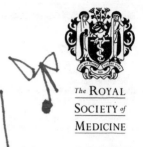

The ROYAL
SOCIETY *of*
MEDICINE

The Royal Society of Medicine (RSM) is an independent medical charity with a primary aim to provide continuing professional development for qualified medical and health-related professionals. The public benefits from health care professionals who have received high quality and relevant education from the RSM.

The Society celebrated its bicentenary in 2005. Each year it arranges and holds over 400 meetings for health care professionals across a wide range of medical subjects. In order to aid education and further training the Society also has the largest postgraduate medical library in Europe – based in central London together with online access to specialist databases. RSM Press, the Society's publishing arm, publishes books and journals principally aimed at the medical profession.

A number of conferences and events are held each year for the public as well as members of the Society. These include the successful 'Medicine and Me' series, designed to bring together patients, their carers and the medical profession. In addition, the RSM's Open and History of Medicine Sections arrange meetings on a regular basis which can be attended by the public.

In addition to the lectures and training provided by the RSM, members of the Society also have access to club facilities including accommodation and a restaurant. The conference and meeting facilities of the RSM were refurbished for their bicentenary and are available to the public for hire for meetings and seminars. In addition, Chandos House, a beautifully restored Georgian townhouse, designed by Robert Adam, is also now available to hire for training, receptions and weddings (as it has a civil wedding licence).

To find out more about the Royal Society of Medicine and the work it undertakes please visit www.rsm.ac.uk or call 020 7290 2991. For more information about RSM Press, please visit www.rsmpress.co.uk.